The Great Pain Jack

A self-help mapping tool to assist you and your physician

in making an accurate diagnosis and appropriate treatment

plan of your chronic or acute pain condition.

by

JOHN F. PETRAGLIA, M.D.

Illustrated by Tanya Hethcoat

authorHOUSE®

AuthorHouse™
1663 Liberty Drive
Bloomington, IN 47403
www.authorhouse.com
Phone: 1-800-839-8640

Published by AuthorHouse 4/20/2012

ISBN: 978-1-4685-6871-4 (sc)
ISBN: 978-1-4685-6870-7 (e)

Library of Congress Control Number: 2012907205

Acknowledgments

This self-help guidebook, *The Great Pain Jack*, is dedicated to my parents, John Sr. and Eleanor, who suffered pain needlessly in their fight against cancer.

To my loving and dedicated wife, Kimberly, and our children, Jordan, Adam, Taylor, Dominic, and Mia, without whom, through their tireless help and encouragement, this book would have never been written.

To those chronic and acute pain sufferers throughout the world who live with pain on a daily basis and to those who have limited understanding of their pain condition and of why they have to suffer. This is my commitment to provide counsel and comfort with honest and valid information to them in their quest for knowledge, education, and relief.

To those who suffer with pain, who take pain medication, although they may not need to, and to those who have been fooled by the inappropriate usage of medication (to those whose brains have been "jacked").

And in memory of James Herold, a creative individual who suffered with chronic pain and passed away before his many earthly talents could fully manifest.

Thank you for being the inspiration to get this book written.

And to Patrick Taylor, a distinguished Army veteran whose indefatigable efforts and valor to analyze, conquer and vanquish chronic pain and headaches have provided new hope and light for other honored serviceman and citizens alike in treatment options for their conditions.

To all my patients, past and present, a huge debt of thanks. By helping you find a way of freeing yourself from chronic pain, I continue to experience again why I chose to be a doctor specializing in this field. I have learned a great deal from your afflictions and will continue to do so as new frontiers of pain open up vistas for new treatment

Contents

Preface

In the age of rationed medical services, with a lack of quality care providers and limited health insurance and access to health care, many pain sufferers do not receive proper medical treatment, or even a proper diagnosis.

After many years of working in the field of pain management, I realized there was an urgent need for a self-help medical guide to help patients, potential patients, and their physicians make accurate diagnoses and employ successful treatment plans for their condition. *The Great Pain Jack* is a statement in and of itself which illustrates how easy an individual can fall victim to misdiagnosis, mismanagement and self- treatment of the pain condition. Without proper therapy and treatment, the brain then becomes potentially "hijacked." "Jack" can be understood to mean a person who has been deluded into thinking that he may be able to treat himself without medical background, and also to suggest a consequence that may occur when the brain is "jacked" under the usage of medication that simply masks symptoms. Please see the website www.gotpaindocs.com, www.thegreatPainJack.com, or www.thegreatPainJack.org for more information.

The book begins with a brief historical overview of pain treatment and continues with a definition of pain and a basic explanation of how the nervous system detects it.

This is followed by a chapter detailing an average day in the life of a pain-management physician, helping you, the patient, understand how a pain doctor thinks and how he or she sees the world. This section deals with everyday medical dramas, battles with health insurance providers, surgical emergencies, and life-or-death situations, as well as the more mundane administrative tasks every pain-management doctor performs daily.

In order to provide specific questions for the area in which you are suffering pain, there are chapters on all parts of the body, beginning with the head and moving through each area of the body. In easy to understand terms, various conditions that can develop and cause pain are discussed together with common treatments for these afflictions. Real-life case studies are woven throughout to illustrate the real-life drama of finding the right diagnosis.

Often patients do not present their physicians with an accurate medical history, or they simply lack the medical knowledge to accurately communicate their symptoms to their doctor. Such misinformation and miscommunication often results in incorrect diagnoses and months, sometimes years, of fruitless trips to various specialists.

For this reason, each chapter in this book ends with a mapping questionnaire intended for you to use so that your physician can better diagnose your affliction and get a good idea of the severity of the pain this affliction is causing. In short, it will help your doctor formulate an appropriate treatment plan.

Without further ado, *The Great Pain Jack* unfolds.

Allow me to work with you to solve your dilemma and support you in discovering, with your physician, a realistic and rational treatment plan for you.

Please refer to the website www.gotpaindocs.com, www.thegreatPainJack.com, or www.thegreatPainJack.org for further information.

Chapter 1:

A Brief History of Pain

Regardless of race, sex, social status, geographical location, and other factors that divide and separate humanity, pain is something we all experience at one point in time. Thus it is no surprise that since the dawn of time humans have invested so much effort into alleviating and treating pain. Pain is not a unique experience only specific to humans.

In almost all of the animal kingdom, we see pain-generating output as a protective mechanism for survival of the species. For example, if a dog is walking with its owner and accidentally crosses its paw under the foot of the dog owner, the dog will let out a yelp and pull its paw away. This is reflexively accomplished within seconds as a protective mechanism for the animal. The next sequence of events (after the dog realizes it is not mortally wounded) may entail that the dog begins to lick its paw. This action then tells the dog's brain that everything is okay and that the "stomp injury" is merely a flesh wound and not something that needs long-term attention. This extremely adaptive yet simple sequence of events is repeated in the animal kingdom often. The message is that the repair or rejuvenation process is already initiated almost at the time of injury, ultimately to shut down the pain signal. This is one example of how the "great pain jack" occurs in nature.

Unsurprisingly the history of pain management goes back to ancient times. A lot of the early pain relief methods involved religious rites, including prayer and exorcism. Egyptians, for instance, thought of manifestations of pain in a person as possession by spirits.

In China a large contribution to medicine was made by Huang Ti, in 2600 BC, who explored the use of acupuncture in pain treatment. The use of opiates such as opium, for example, due to their anesthetic properties, goes back to ancient times as well, with uses documented in the Trojan Wars in 1220 BC.

Hippocrates, a Greek after whom the Hippocratic Oath is named, focused not on the disease but on the patient—a focus that is prevalent in modern chronic pain treatment. All medical students take the Hippocratic Oath and commit to doing "no harm," though in many chronic pain treatments the opposite can seem to be the case from the patient's point of view.

During the Middle Ages, many of the texts documenting advances in pain management made by the Greeks and Romans were buried and/or destroyed in Europe. However, medical studies flourished in the Middle East, where some of these texts were preserved. During the Renaissance, many of these texts resurfaced in Europe.

Opium was a popular prescription form of pain relief until it was diluted into laudanum, a painkiller used until well into the nineteenth century. Also, during the eighteenth and nineteenth centuries, major leaps were made in reducing pain during limb surgery, resulting in the use of cocaine as an anesthetic. In 1817 pharmacist F. W. A. Serturner made a significant contribution to pain management by creating morphine.

Ether was introduced as an anesthetic in surgery, and by the end of the nineteenth century it was replaced by chloroform. Karl Koller, an Austrian ophthalmologist, explored the numbing effects of cocaine, which led him to discover local anesthesia; that is, instead of the patient going under completely, only the region in need of treatment could be numbed. Koller's contribution to pain treatment was revolutionary and paved the way for the emergence of nerve-block techniques and other modern pain treatment methods.

The twentieth century is marked by many significant medical discoveries and inventions with the sole goal of preserving life and easing pain. Sir Alexander Fleming's discovery of penicillin in 1928, John Hopps's invention of the pacemaker in 1950, Willem J. Kolff's invention of the artificial heart, and the invention of HIV protease inhibitors in the late 1980s and early 1990s, as well as recent advances in genetic engineering and stem cell research, are all milestones in pain management.

Despite all these advances, millions of people all over the world experience acute and chronic pain every year. Their lives often take the form of a struggle from one day to the next, with no hope of relief in sight. Modern medicine has solutions for many of them, but these solutions are useless without a proper diagnosis. The case studies and analyses in this book stress the importance of accurate diagnoses in successful pain-management treatment. If the correct diagnosis and proper treatment is not initiated, "the great pain jack" may be initiated.

Chapter 2:

Definition and Types of Pain

L et us begin with a definition of *pain*. The IASP (International Society for the Study of Pain) defines pain as: "*an unpleasant sensory and emotional experience associated with actual or potential tissue damage, or described in terms of such damage.*"

The note at the end of the definition goes on to say that pain "is always subjective." Pain can also exist in the absence of tissue damage, where it takes a psychological form. This book will focus almost entirely on physical pain, though I do use the expertise of a psychologist specializing in "psychological aspects of pain" as part of my treatment team. The mind can often be stronger than the body, and research is bringing new insights into the role of mind over matter.

Physical pain, especially when severe, will often have a serious psychological component and certainly serious mental health issues, not the least of which is dependence, which can arise from untreated and chronic physical pain. For instance, surgery for a defect causing abdominal tissues to descend into the groin area, known as inguinal hernia, may result in a condition called "nerve entrapment." Consequently, pain may develop in the groin area, affecting the sufferer's sexual life and his family life, and in general, result in depression. If the necessary surgery to repair the condition is not preformed, the condition may worsen and lead to other complications.

Pain may be subdivided into a number of different categories. For example there is somatic pain, neuropathic pain, visceral pain, nociceptive pain, arthritic pain, pain from cancer, sympathetic mediated pain, nerve damage pain, mixed pain, and psychogenic pain.

Pain becomes chronic when it persists for more than three to six months. It is important to realize that chronic pain may be caused by an anatomical or correctable medical problem. The problem, when undiagnosed or untreated, may become chronic and cause additional types of pain, which may be worse than the original condition. An example would be the care of an inguinal hernia repair, which then could be complicated by the entrapment of small nerve fibers in repair mesh. The resulting condition is known as ilioinguinal neuralgia.

Case Study: Bob, a young painter and plaster handyman, fell off a scaffold and broke a small bone in his wrist. The bone, however, did not heal properly. Since the pain would not go away, Bob went to see his doctor. The doctor examined his hand carefully and found it necessary to perform a surgical procedure known as open reduction and internal fixation.

Yet, after the surgery, Bob continued to experience pain in his hand. In fact, the condition worsened, and, over a brief period of time, he lost all functionality in it. A complex regional pain syndrome developed in his appendage, and Bob was forced to go through several other surgeries as a result. While the fracture finally healed, the failure did not heal in a timely and normal fashion. This activated the nerves of the sympathetic nervous system and caused more damage. Bob developed severe limb and spinal problems that necessitated painful, extremely complex surgical procedures to treat.

Bob's story weighs on every doctor's mind, reminding us how crucial an early, correct diagnosis truly is. If Bob's condition had been diagnosed earlier, many of the aforementioned problems would have never occurred.

Of course, diseases and medical conditions don't always allow for an easy diagnosis. Many are discovered over long periods of time, after a series of tests, guesses, and experiments. This book will offer tools that attempt to lessen the time between the manifestation of a disease or condition and its accurate diagnosis, by education of the patient about pain and by how to communicate this information most accurately to one's doctor.

In the forthcoming chapters, we will journey through the body, beginning with the head, and address some of the more common problems, diseases, and syndromes that can arise, as well as the various treatments available to combat them. I will touch on the unusual and some uncommon pain syndromes and their treatments as well. More information may be obtained from the website www.gotpaindocs.com, www.ThegreatPainJack.com, or www.ThegreatPainJack.org for specific treatment of complex regional pain syndrome.

It is always important to remember that pain is a signal that something is wrong. It is the body attempting to give us some crucial, and in many cases "lifesaving," information. Numbing it with drugs or pills or in any other way can obscure the cause of the pain. The idea is always to manage the pain while finding out the underlying cause or causes in order that the root of the pain can be discovered and treated.

Chapter 3:

Introduction to a World of Pain

I t's 5:40 a.m. on a Tuesday. I've already reviewed the day's agenda, which was culled from three days' worth of operative reports and office notes securely forwarded to me via Internet and e-mail. Despite the average four and a half hours of sleep, I feel quite energetic.

Even with the morning's preparation, the day has its share of surprises. I arrive at the pain management clinic at 8:00 a.m., and sure enough, I am informed that an emergency lumbar epidural steroid injection has been added to my schedule. The patient is now in the waiting room, nervously pacing in pain.

The phone starts ringing, and it will not stop. Today calls are being forwarded from two other office locations; the usual call volume is magnified. A patient with excruciating, steadily worsening back pain is asking for more Percocet. A hospital calls requesting an "emergency consult" for an unfortunate individual with an undefined pain phenomenon, who was admitted in the last twenty-four hours. A slew of ER and family physicians, neurologists, orthopedic surgeons, and other specialists are already debating how to help this patient. If the patient is already taking strong medication for his pain, like OxyContin or morphine, that usually triggers a call to me, a pain management physician.

While still on the line with the hospital, I get a call from another hospital about a patient in the emergency room with redness and drainage from his morphine pump implant site, placed one week ago.

Meanwhile, another patient is waiting for me in exam room one. Accompanied by his insurance company case manager, he wants to discuss the quantity of Vicodin pills that he should take for a minor work-related injury. He's been directed to me by his attorney because both his employer and his workers' compensation carrier do not believe that he is truly injured. His colleague ran over his foot with a fork lift, and he lost two and a half of his toes. He now has a substantial injury with a condition known as complex regional pain disorder of the lower extremity. The employer wants to know why this individual can't go back to work since his condition has improved (after amputation of the toes) and over eight months have passed since the injury. Another "great pain jack."

The gentleman in exam room two has run out of the OxyContin prescribed by his previous physician and is here for another dose recommendation. He was referred to me after being released by his doctor for "dereliction of duty" and failure to read the fine print of the narcotics agreement, which states that "under no circumstances can a person receiving prescription medication, intake any illicit or nonprescribed medication or medication of the same type prescribed at the same time by another physician into the body." Another victim of "the great pain jack."

As I pass by the exam room I pick up the strong, distinct smell of tobacco and marijuana. While he did not smoke in the exam room, I often find patients who have used nonprescription drugs before seeing their doctor, especially after running out of their regular prescription medication. Pain can be unforgiving. Dependence can be unrelenting. Addiction can be deadly. Chronic pain can really "jack" you and your brain

The operating room calls to let me know that the emergency lumbar epidural steroid injection patient is prepped, draped, and ready for her lumbar epidural and sacroiliac joint injections. I perform them. I finish the procedure. When I leave the operating room, I learn from my office manager that Medicare has requested fifteen charts for medical review and is threatening an audit if they do not receive the information by the end of the week.

I am stopped from attending my next appointment by a call from a doctor regarding a request for a radiofrequency nerve ablation (a treatment for spine pain) for a patient. I begin to feel slight withdrawal from the coffee I badly need; I try to persuade the doctor, who works for the patient's insurance company, that the procedure is necessary for her well-being. The smell of coffee from our kitchen seems awfully tempting!

My other office calls and informs me that the local police department has referred a patient on an urgent basis who held up a pharmacy using a utility belt tool. Apparently they needed the person evaluated on a timely basis because after holding up the pharmacy (while using a wrench) and succeeding, he ingested a large quantity of narcotic medications formulated into a patch. After becoming immediately intoxicated with the box of ingested narcotic patches, he managed to crash his vehicle into a utility pole. The police then rounded him up and pressed charges. He pleaded the "fentanyl frenzy" defense for his crime while undergoing treatment of an existing medical condition.

Sadly, this individual, who had clearly been "hijacked" by pain and addiction, was found dead two weeks later. Another somber, late "great pain jack."

The telephone conversation with the doctor that wants to disapprove of the radiofrequency ablation of the spine gets a little heated; the doctor clearly has not read the detailed reports I sent him along with my treatment-authorization request. It doesn't help that his mission is to turn down my request since his goal is to "preserve" the insurance company's money. In the end, he assures me that he will submit his report to the carrier and, in a routine maneuver, and pleasantly, reminds me of my right to appeal the carrier's decision.

While some doctors can be reasonable, the majority of these conversations can get very hostile and tense. It's easy to get caught up in the uphill battle that unravels regarding treatment plans over the phone with insurance companies. This is another example of the physician's version of "the great pain jack." Often, I want to simply give up. However, it's difficult to overstate the fact that often lives and well-beings are literally at stake during such talks. So when a report comes back to me classifying a necessary procedure as "noncertified," I have to prepare for verbal battle. It's part of my job and my duty to my patients. Such combat takes skill, nuance, tact, and persistence. You have to pick your fights well. You have to know when to hold or when to fold, and when to persist. And the good doctor will be hearing from me. It's a bit like poker in that sense.

I look at my watch. It's only 9:10 a.m. A medical assistant informs me that a well-known national insurance company is refusing to authorize a neural stimulator trial for a chronic pain patient, a possible life-changing treatment for this individual. I decide to return to this later and head for the operating room.

There I greet a patient of mine who has survived facial cancer. Unfortunately, the radiation treatments have left his neck, face, and spine in a distorted state. Our eyes meet and a broad smile comes across his face. I smile back at this calm but spirited seventy-six-year-old man and chat with him as I provide an anesthetic through an IV. Quickly, it takes effect. His eyes close.

I can sense the radiation-induced tension in his muscles subside. I perform a cervical epidural injection and, using a fluoroscope (a real-time x-ray machine), I watch the infused dye enter the cervical nerve roots of the epidural space. I now inject an anesthetic steroid, the drug that will keep my friend and patient off all of his pain medications for two to three months. His aged body does not tolerate pain medications very well.

The dye material dissipates with my second booster cocktail injection of anesthetic mixed with a steroid. The fifteen-minute procedure will save the patient from surgery. I may perform eight to twelve such injections on a daily basis.

After the procedure, my friend bids me good-bye and leaves with that smile on his face I've come to know well. I've seen it on the face of the woman who experienced relief from her postherpetic neuralgia for the first time in five years after an epidural injection. Or the boy who finally got his pain pump implanted. Or Mrs. B———, who, nearly driven to suicide by pain from three failed back surgeries, finally received a neural stimulator implant that gave her a new lease on life.

Unfortunately, many stories don't always come with happy endings. There are the occasional calls from coroners' offices and family members questioning the use of strong medications to control pain. With the number of accidental overdoses related to prescription drugs experientially on the rise in the last decade, these types of phone calls will naturally be more frequent to physician offices. However, an interventional pain management physician is in a unique position to help some of the most desperate patients. He or she has the specialized knowledge, resources, and technical expertise to perform modern-day medical miracles, improving the quality of life for chronic and acute pain sufferers immensely.

In the end, the greatest joy and biggest satisfaction is witnessing the patients' relief from pain. It is hard to fully appreciate it from outside the doctor's office, but one has to remember that a lot of the people who come to see me often suffer from severe, at times excruciating, pain that has plagued them for several years. It disrupts their daily lives. It prevents them from enjoying simple physical activities like walking, eating, shopping, and bathing. It affects them emotionally and psychologically. It depresses and destroys the very essence of their lives. Recovery for a lot of these patients is a sacred event, a kind of rebirth. I take great pride in being a part of it.

Finally at 8:00 p.m. I head home. Trying to find a balance in one's own life for family and recreation isn't easy. I finish going through my e-mail, sending directions regarding management of patients at remote office locations, responding to new pain management queries solicited from the Internet, updating a mandated electronic medical file on hundreds of patients, and finalizing surgical scheduling for the next five days. Then, I go to sleep.

Chapter 4:

Dependence, Addiction, Tolerance, and Pseudoaddiction

What do Anna Nicole Smith, Michael Jackson, Danny Gans, Elvis Presley, River Phoenix, and Heath Ledger have in common? They all died of accidental poisoning due to combinations of prescription painkillers and other intoxicating substances. Death from "accidental poisonings," the medical term for intentional or unintentional overdose, has dramatically increased in the last decade. These accidental deaths are in part due to the ubiquitous availability of prescription painkillers, narcotics, tranquilizers, and antianxiety medications. The trend toward ready and formidable treatment of pain with opioid medication has played a role in this trend. The high availability and sense of "legality" associated with these prescription meds because they are prescribed by a doctor has lowered the threshold for caution for their "routine" use by many individuals.

When these medications are taken in combination (appropriately or inappropriately prescribed), the results can be disastrous. In the case of the above celebrity examples, doctors are often afraid to clamp down on improper use of these types of medications by their recipients. However, they can be held accountable for their prescription writing carelessness, especially to people with dependency addiction concerns or emotional instability issues.

With a new prescription medication, a follow-up with the patient is absolutely imperative to assess the drug's effect on neurological and respiratory functions, as well as the efficacy of dosing of the drug. Medications like Demerol, morphine, OxyContin, and long-acting variations of these medications may be prescribed for treating chronic pain. When combinations of classes of medications, including antianxiety pills, major tranquilizers, sleeping pills, and muscle relaxants, are combined with narcotic analgesics, their effects may be lethal, as in the case of some of the celebrity examples listed above.

Narcotic analgesics such as morphine block pain receptors in the body and act on specific opioid receptors to produce a numbing, euphoric feeling. Most of the receptors are in the brain and spinal cord. The body's own natural equivalent to these narcotic analgesics is the class of chemicals known as endorphins. Endorphins are protein molecules the body releases to promote a feeling of "*well-being*," for example after vigorous exercise, alcohol consumption, or sexual activity. They circulate through the body and bind to opioid receptors, which stimulate the aforementioned feeling. Thus, when runners talk about the "runner's high," they are actually referring to the release of endorphins during their run and to the positive effect of the natural chemicals on the body.

An understanding of the terms *dependence, tolerance, addiction* and *pseudoaddiction* is important in understanding the body's ability to process these medications. Physical dependence and tolerance are both natural consequences of extended opioid therapy for pain. *Dependence* is a physiological state in which the abrupt cessation or dose reduction results in withdrawal in the patient. *Tolerance* occurs when the body begins to require an increasing or more frequent dosage to produce a specific effect, i.e., both the analgesic (pain-relieving effect) and the side effects of the medications. These terms elucidate and are examples of how "the great pain jack" can literally take over control of one's life.

> **Case Study:** *A young, professional, and clean-cut man, Mr. C———, once came to see me complaining of lower back and shoulder pain. C, aside from being a very successful currency and stock trader, was also an avid bodybuilder, which probably contributed to some of his pain through injury.*
>
> *He had been prescribed OxyContin for the pain by another doctor. However, he had upped his intake from two to four times a day, explaining that he needed at least two pills for his regular extensive morning workout. This drug-fueled routine went on for a few months. Mr. C——— seemed to require more and more medication to obtain the same measure of relief. In other words, he developed a tolerance to his medication.*
>
> *During the course of our discussion, C——— admitted that he was now taking up to twelve to fourteen 80 mg OxyContin tablets a day. This shocked me. I could not believe this man was ingesting 960 mg of OxyContin on a daily basis for what was probably the better part of six to nine months. Moreover, it was obvious that he was getting the additional eight pills a day from another source. Needless to say, an OxyContin addiction, aside from being dangerous, is an expensive habit.*
>
> *As this information unraveled, C——— told me that he wanted to stop taking the medication but couldn't. He needed it now just to get up in the morning, to do his daily exercise routine, and to perform other, basic tasks. It wasn't long before C——— stopped feeling pain altogether. This can be a very serious condition. People who take large quantities of narcotics and stop feeling pain can often injure themselves without realizing it. Indeed, there are many documented instances of patients under the heavy influence of drugs who have burned themselves on the stove or cut their hands on glass and been unaware of it. The analgesic effect of the medication was obliterating even normal, necessary warning signs.*

C—— said he wanted to try a detoxification program. As a first step, for a month I cut his OxyContin dose down to one-third of what it was. The following month, I started him on suboxone therapy, which involves taking opioid antagonist medication, a narcotic, to help the patient come off his or her drug addiction. And a month after that C—— stopped taking OxyContin altogether. For now at least, he was in the clear, off the pain medication and working with a treatment plan to deal with his pain. His switching to a different medication has not been completely successful in ridding his desire to continue taking his first-choice medication. He continues to undergo treatment with our pain physiologist and addictionalogist.

Of course, not all detoxification programs are successful. Detoxification works best if the addict, like Mr. C——, displays extreme desire and willpower to overcome his or her addiction.

Addiction is characterized by substance craving, as well as compulsive and continued use despite harmful consequences. Often illegal, indications of bizarre behavior may be evident.

> **Addiction Case Study:** *Mary is a twenty-seven-year-old woman who complained of chronic pain due to a car accident. I took a thorough look at her medical history and performed a physical exam. It soon became clear that she did not have a detectable pain syndrome, at least not anymore. I began to suspect an addiction problem. I suspected a "pain jacking."*
>
> *After some prodding, the patient admitted that after the accident she began seeing a chiropractor, and her overall condition improved. About a year ago, after the chiropractic sessions ended, she saw her former physician, who prescribed her for pain, for no apparent reason, 80 mg OxyContin to take twice a day.*
>
> *Over time, the woman upped her dosage from two to five tablets a day, without the consent of her physician. She tried to wean herself off the medication but slowly began to realize that the condition was beyond her control. She was addicted, and the addiction began to take over her life and her daily activities. Eureka, bull's-eye!! Another "great pain jacking" discovered.*
>
> *After our conversation, Mary signed up for a detoxification program at my office, and, as of the time of writing of this book, she has completed the treatment plan with excellent results. She has begun studies to become a physician's assistant, and she no longer has a medication dependency.*

The lesson is that potent narcotic medication has very seductive qualities, which a patient may desire long after the chronic pain condition has been resolved. Thus in the process of getting better, the brain get "jacked" and then doesn't want to have anything to do with other necessary ingredients of remedy. Please see www.thegreatPainJack.com for more information.

Pseudoaddiction occurs when a patient's pain is undertreated. As a result patients may exhibit addictive behaviors in order to obtain additional pain-relief medication. For instance, a person prescribed opioids (painkillers, such as morphine, that act on opioid receptors) for chronic pain syndrome may be doing well with a specific dosage for the first few weeks or months.

It is the case, though, that the condition may change, such as the demands of physical therapy, new job, life stressors, or an additional new injury, etc., and may well increase the body's need for a higher dosage. The patient's doctor may be reluctant to increase the dosage, being unable to account for the need. Pseudoaddiction manifests itself when the patient goes to the emergency room for a shot, for example, or begins to seek the medications from others. However, if the increased dosage is prescribed, the pseudoaddiction behaviors end as well, unlike with addiction. The pain is actually undertreated with pseudoaddiction.

Dosing of Medications

More than seventy-five million Americans are estimated to suffer from severe chronic pain each year. For many patients, opioid analgesics are the only treatment option that provides significant relief. Preventing abuse is an important aspect of pain management but should not interfere with the patient's ability to receive appropriate treatment. The World Health Organization uses a three-step ladder to direct the use of pain medication:

> *Step 1 (mild pain)—the use of nonopioids such as aspirin or nonsteroidal anti-inflammatory drugs is recommended.*

> *Step 2 (mild to moderate pain)—the use of less-intensive opioids such as codeine or hydrocodone is recommended.*

> *Step 3 (moderate to severe pain)—the use of stronger opioids such as morphine, hydromorphone, or oxycodone is recommended.*

The dose varies widely among patients, and it is based on maximizing pain relief and limiting side effects experienced by the patient. Long-term therapy is typically started at a low dose and raised until an adequate level of pain relief is reached or side effects become difficult to contain or manage. If pain persists throughout the day, analgesics should be administered on a scheduled, consistent basis to keep the flow of medication in the bloodstream constant. Long-acting opioids are generally best suited for patients with chronic pain. For elderly patients, the dosage may be reduced up to 25 to 50 percent as compared to that of younger patients because the elderly may be more susceptible to the adverse effects of opioid medications.

When a person comes into the office and says that he or she has been prescribed an opioid medication by another doctor and requests a refill, the patient immediately raises a red flag to me and my staff. Why is this individual seeking medication from a second physician? The common response "I just moved from another area" could be true but usually raises concern. On the other hand, when it is genuine, and the need is there for the prescription, the patient may go into withdrawal without a refill. Sometimes patients will ask for more pills than necessary to avoid getting their medication filled on a monthly basis. For some it is a matter of economics or a lack of understanding that medication is usually filled on a monthly basis. Others will ask for more pills in an effort to distribute them illegally. Such is often the case with frequent travelers, who sell or take medications in different cities. One concern of local high schools is that the medications obtained illegally will serve as a barter mechanism or "currency" in the schools. This is another primary example in modern society of "the great pain jack."

A physician must weigh such factors every day when deciding whether to prescribe medication to a patient, up the dosage, or refuse to renew a prescription. Each of these decisions carries with it huge consequences, and therefore extreme care must be undertaken when making them. He must resist "the great pain jack."

Case Study: A young Asian American male, Yu, came to see me and told me that he developed back and neck pain as a result of a car accident he was involved in two years earlier. Visits to a chiropractor provided temporary relief, but eventually his pain became chronic, and there was nothing the chiropractor could do.

I asked Yu if he had x-rays or an MRI performed on his back and neck. He said that he hadn't. I began to suspect something was suspicious since x-rays or MRI studies are a standard procedure after a motor vehicle accident, no matter how minor it may be.

When Yu said he took eight OxyContin 80 mg tablets a day, my suspicions were confirmed. I did not believe that his medication was legitimately prescribed. After examining him, I believed he did not need even one pill a day. Yu did not like what I told him and tried bargaining with me for a prescription of at least six pills per day. I refused.

After a long conversation with him, I reviewed the signs and symptoms of his condition and also asked what his last dose of medication was. We settled on two OxyContin tablets a day for two weeks to keep him from going into withdrawal. I reasoned that if he was legitimately seeking drugs for pain he would return after the two weeks.

I never saw him again.

Side Effects of Medication and Withdrawal

Common side effects of opioid analgesics include constipation, sedation, nausea, vomiting, itching, confusion, and difficulty breathing. Though patients generally develop a tolerance to these side effects, a doctor should monitor them. The main exception is constipation;

if undergoing opioid therapy for the first time, a patient should receive stool softeners or medication to increase bowel movements.

Breathing problems resulting from these medications generally occur only in patients new to opioids or to those who mix them with other substances. The difficulty breathing, notably the slowing respiratory rate effect, is specific to narcotic analgesics. Our bodies have a control mechanism that ensures that we keep on breathing. This respiratory drive is stimulated by chemical receptors deep within the brain. Narcotic analgesics all typically allow a higher amount of carbon dioxide to enter the bloodstream before the breathing response kicks in.

Dangerous combinations of cocktails including alcohol, tranquilizers, or sleeping pills taken in combination with regular prescription painkillers may so significantly blunt the respiratory drive mechanism that the patient may suffer respiratory depression, brain damage, or premature death. For those reasons, physicians and painkiller labels warn against alcohol use when taking prescription opioid analgesics. However, when medications are dosed and monitored appropriately, respiratory depression is uncommon.

Case Study: Dylan, a stocky and heavy twenty-year-old, came to see me regarding pain in his lower back. When in high school, he played football and got a herniated disk in his back. At age eighteen, Dylan underwent a diskectomy and fusion surgery, convinced by his doctor that this would make his pain go away.

The surgery went well, and Dylan was pain-free. However, for whatever reason, within six months of the surgery he developed recurrent back pain. He began taking medication, which gradually increased in intensity and dosage, for the pain. He was now taking large, around-the-clock doses of methadone, morphine, and OxyContin to control symptoms. Dylan's burning need for drugs steadily escalated, and at the ripe age of twenty Dylan began shooting heroin into his veins.

Soon, his drug addiction led to altercations with gang members and drug dealers, ultimately resulting in assault charges alleged against him. The first day I met him, I asked him when he last took any prescribed medication or recreational drugs. He shot me a blank stare and said he injected heroin the day before. I studied this clean-cut, former high school football star from a well-to-do, high-income neighborhood and digested this information. I hoped Dylan was reaching out for help.

I was trying to determine if he was going through any withdrawal symptoms such as agitation, high blood pressure and pulse rate, goose bumps, nausea, and vomiting. I needed to also check Dylan for any number of related conditions such as infection, neurologic impairment, cardiovascular risk, stroke, etc. Finally, I had to decide on how to go about treating him. We screened his urine that day for verification of his facts. His urine proved positive for a number of illicit substances, some prescribed, some not.

I thanked Dylan for his honesty, praising his decision to seek professional help. I counseled him about the dangers of continued use of street and prescription drugs, such as overdose, respiratory depression, death, heart attack, and brain injury. Dylan was eager to get help. He signed an opioid agreement, requiring him to be monitored on a weekly basis.

I prescribed him small doses of Xanax to ease his withdrawal symptoms. For physical pain, he was only allowed to take ibuprofen or nonsteroidal anti-inflammatory medication. With the help of Narcotics Anonymous, Dylan would be subjected to strict urine testing and peer group counseling. This was supplemented by in-office urine tests and a written pledge to sobriety.

I will never know why Dylan decided to seek help that day—maybe he had had a bad trip, or simply began to realize the toll drugs were taking on his life—but I know he was serious about getting sober. After his first, brutally honest, drug therapy session, he began his detoxification program, and, as of the writing of this book, he has remained sober.

Urine testing is often provided in pain management clinics to make sure that only prescribed medication is contained within the urine and nothing else. The practice has become very commonplace and is a very good indicator of what medications a patient has taken over a three-day period.

The Drug Enforcement Agency is seeking ways to limit the illegitimate use of medications. For example, one strategy involves prescribing a narcotic that has another prescription painkiller contained within it. If the outer narcotic is crushed, smoked, or taken in a manner other than intended, the inner compound becomes active and prevents the euphoric effect of the narcotic. This medication has been prescribed and used with moderate effectiveness.

In another, more long-term, effort, the federal government mandates that pain management clinics develop REMS or Risk Evaluation Management Strategy. These systems allow physicians to classify patients as high, medium, or low risk for drug abuse. The clinic is solely responsible for these classifications and for taking action with high-risk individuals, especially those who have demonstrated red-flag behaviors. This may include dismissal from the clinic, a more intense evaluation with history and physical exam, entry into a detoxification program, or counseling. If a patient is proven to abuse his or her medication and divert medication away for whatever reason, the clinic may be held responsible. A local newspaper championed the raiding and closure of another pain clinic that had prescribed medication to a teenager. Apparently the teenager sold or gave some of the medication to another teenager, who unfortunately overdosed and died. The doctor of the clinic said publicly, "I did nothing wrong." The case, among others, is currently being reviewed.

Nevertheless, an increasing number of deaths are attributed to improper use of narcotic analgesics. Therefore, it is extremely important for patients to comply with their doctors' recommendations when taking medication for chronic pain. While it is absolutely normal for a sufferer to seek pain relief, recreational use of painkillers may have devastating results for both the patient and the physician. The consequences of an unintentional death could involve manslaughter charges and possibly even murder charges against doctors that have prescribed these medications. The main problem, however, is the growing black market for these types of prescription medications. As a result, many lawsuits target traffickers and pain clinics that provide these potent narcotics to individuals who claim they need the medications.

The routine use of prescription painkillers and their widespread use in our society to treat painful conditions has exploded. Without proper monitoring, dose adjustment, and strict enforcement of individual use, overdoses associated with such medications will continue to increase.

Case Study: I met Travis on a very busy day. Patients were coming in and out of the clinic in rapid succession, yet Travis completely stood out. The reason was simple. When he met me, he told me he had broken thirty-one bones in his body, and he wanted something for the pain. He was only twenty-two years old.

Travis was a motocross rider who performed death-defying jumps and stunts, and participated in motorcycle races and motorcycle stunts. While I could see he reflected his age in his love of living on the edge, I could not understand the attraction to his crazy job.

Getting into the mind of a twenty-two-year-old who lives for the gravity-defying stunts of the motocross rider, risking his life on a daily basis, can be a difficult thing to do. I was at first hesitant to prescribe him any medication, fearing that he might be an adrenaline junkie. Prescribing narcotic painkillers to an adrenaline junkie might lead to more dangerous behavior, including a drug-fueled feeling of invincibility.

I didn't want to put Travis in a situation where he would put himself at more risk than he already has because of medication I prescribed. Travis, however, assured me that he only took medication after his rides. He provided me with reports of his emergency room visits due to his broken bones and other trauma. He promised me, almost gleefully watching my reaction, that he would continue to ride regardless of the hazard to his health.

I explained the effects of long-term use of narcotics, anti-inflammatories and muscle relaxants on his gastrointestinal, hormone, and sexual functions, but none of this seemed to scare him. If he jumped dozens of feet in the air on a motorcycle, he also knew the dangers of drug abuse. I could see if I didn't prescribe the medication for him, he would get them from somewhere else.

I weighed my options for him and decided on a controlled time-release analgesic and anti-inflammatory regimen for his multiple joint pain conditions and likely early arthritis. In exchange, he agreed to obtain his medication from only one doctor and from only one pharmacy and to take them as prescribed. He agreed to return if the pills did not ease his pain or if the symptoms became so difficult to manage that the prescription might need to be changed. He thanked me and left.

A few weeks later he returned. He brought me beautiful glossy pictures and videos of his performance on the motocross track. I thanked him, astounded by both his bravery and lunacy.

I know Travis will return as his arthritis worsens, and unfortunately he may need complex chronic pain management in his later years. Please refer to the websites www.gotpaindocs. com, www.thegreatPainJack.com, or www.thegreatPainJack.org for further information.

John F. Petraglia, M.D.

Screening tool to help you and your doctor identify relative risk for both of you with respect to prescribed medication

This "Use" questionnaire is one tool to help doctors and their patients in an effort to help determine how much monitoring a patient on long -term pain therapy may ultimately require . Physicians often remain reluctant to prescribe pain medication because of concerns about addiction, misuse, dependency, overdose as well as liability concerns. This factor may be more pronounced when dealing with certain ages and populations due to existing natural prejudices. Some studies suggest that patients are successfully able to remain on long-term pain therapy without significant problems. However, physicians often do not have the skill set or staff to determine the relative risk for developing problems when their patients are placed on long -term pain therapy.

Answer the questions on the test if you are already taking or being considered for prescription opioid medication to treat chronic pain. Please answer each question honestly.

Please answer the questions below using the following scale:

0 = Never, 1 = Rarely 2 = Sometimes 3 = Often 4 = Almost every day

1. How often have you felt a desire or deep craving for medication?   0   1   2   3   4

2. How often do you have mood swings?   0   1   2   3   4

3. How often do you smoke a cigarette within an hour after you wake up?   0   1   2   3   4

4. How often / have any family members, including parents and grandparents, had a problem with alcohol or drugs?   0   1   2   3   4

5. How often have any of your close friends had a problem with alcohol or drugs?   0   1   2   3   4

6. How often have others suggested that you have a drug or alcohol problem?   0   1   2   3   4

7. How often have you attended an AA or NA meeting?   0   1   2   3   4

8. How often have you taken medication other than the way it was prescribed (route of admin. or frequency of taking the med ?)   0   1   2   3   4

9. How often have you been treated for an alcohol or drug problem?   0   1   2   3   4

10. How often have your medications been lost, stolen or "disappeared"?   0   1   2   3   4

11. How often have others expressed concern over your use of medication?   0   1   2   3   4

12. How often have you been asked to give a urine screen at work   0   1   2   3   4
or school for substance abuse?

13. How often have you used illegal drugs (for example, marijuana,   0   1   2   3   4
cocaine, etc.) in the past five years?

14. How often, in your lifetime, have you had legal problems or   0   1   2   3   4
been arrested?

Scoring Instructions for the "Use" questionnaire

To score the test, simply add the ratings of all the questions: A score of 7.5 or higher is considered positive. For any screening test, the results depend on what cutoff score is chosen. A score that is good at detecting patients at-risk will, by design include a number of patients that are not really at risk at all . A score that is excellent at identifying low risk will, in turn, miss a number of patients at risk. A screening tool such as the questionnaire will strive to minimize the chances of missing high-risk individuals. This means that patients who appear to be at low risk may receive a score above the cutoff. The data suggest that the "Use" questionnaire is a sensitive test. This confirms that the "Use" questionnaire is better at identifying high risk individuals than identifying low risk individuals.

Chapter 5:

So, You've Got Headache Pain?

Arteriovenous Malformation: *Celeste, a forty-four-year-old woman with a severe history of migraine headaches, came to see me. She told me she had recently fallen, fractured her ribs, and got a large contusion under her right breast. On top of that, her headaches grew more severe with each day since the accident.*

What was truly amazing about Celeste was that she had a condition known as arteriovenous malformation in her brain, diagnosed some twenty years prior. She was even considered for brain surgery at the time, using a computer assisted gamma knife, a type of high-tech neurosurgery without a scalpel. The surgery basically targets areas in the brain using computer-assisted guidance. She apparently refused to go through with the procedure, believing it wasn't necessity.

I asked Celeste why she didn't follow up with the neurologist who initially diagnosed her. She almost blithely told me that she didn't think it was important. I asked her if she remembered the symptoms she had when she was initially diagnosed twenty years ago. She said they were similar to her current ones. She would get daily headaches, lose her appetite, get blurry vision, her eyeballs hurt, and she would occasionally lose her balance.

It seemed to me that she did not want to face her condition by avoiding a follow up with the doctors who had made the diagnosis two decades earlier. Could her brain have been "hijacked?" Instead, she had been medicating herself with different painkillers that she very likely got from the street, since she had no prescription to show for them. She also didn't have health insurance, and so she could not easily get prescriptions, much less visit a doctor.

I promptly requested her old medical records and received minimal notes. I referred her to a neurologist regarding her arteriovenous malformation, as the condition could kill her. It is something some of us are born with, and it becomes a problem if bleeding or rupture occurs in the brain, or if the malformation presses on vital brain structures. Her symptoms seemed to indicate an imminent rupture. I prescribed an intercostal block injection for her fractured ribs. I have little confidence she will treat this serious condition with the attention it deserves, but it will undoubtedly get her attention in a dramatic way at some point.

Among the various types of headaches, the most common include migraines, tension-type headaches, cluster headaches, headaches due to acute herpes zoster of the first division of the trigeminal nerve, medication rebound headaches, and headaches due to occipital neuralgia. Please refer to the website www.gotpaindocs.com, www.thegreatPainJack.com, or www.thegreatPainJack.org for further information.

Migraines

A migraine, one of the most common headaches, almost always develops in a person before the age of thirty. Migraine attacks vary in frequency from one every few days to once every few months. Approximately 65 percent of the sufferers are females, and many report a family history of migraines. People who get migraines tend to fit a certain psychological profile. They are often characterized as neat, meticulous, and compulsive. They typically tend to be excessive in their daily habits and have coping difficulty with everyday life stresses. Some of the more common migraine triggers include changes in sleep patterns or diet, ingestion of chocolate or citrus fruits, and changes in hormone levels such as those resulting from the use of birth control pills.

Approximately 20 percent of patients who suffer from migraines often experience a painless neurologic event before the beginning of the headache, which is called an *aura*. The aura most often manifests itself as a visual disturbance, but also may present itself as an alteration in smell or hearing. It is thought to be caused by a lack of blood supply to specific regions of the cerebral cortex. Visual aura will often occur thirty to sixty minutes before the migraine and may take the form of blind spots called *scotomas*, which are essentially flashing zigzag disruptions of vision.

Occasionally, migraine patients may lose their entire visual field. Auditory auras include hypersensitivity to sound, as well as perceiving sounds of objects as farther than they actually are. Olfactory aura, equally, may take the form of extreme hypersensitivity to normal odors or the sensation of odors not actually emitted by anything. Occasionally, a migraine sufferer might experience a prolonged neurologic dysfunction, which can last more than twenty-four hours and is called *migraine with prolonged aura*. This may take the form of one-sided weakness of the body, or speech impairment or loss.

Although with each episode the headache may switch sides, migraines never occur on both sides of the head at the same time. The pain is usually focused around or behind the eye. It is typically pounding in nature, its intensity is severe, and it may be accompanied by nausea, vomiting, photophobia (fear of looking at lights), sonophobia (fear of sounds), and changes in appetite, mood, or libido.

Case Study: A lot of migraine sufferers who come to see me often wear sunglasses to keep the sun out of their eyes. When they slink into the exam room, they request the lights be turned off. A particular patient of mine, Lorraine, comes to mind. She worked as a defense attorney and suffered migraines almost her whole life. The condition interfered tremendously with her work and cut down on her quality family time. I treated her by combining medications with occipital nerve blocks to reduce greatly the severity and frequency of the headaches. Please see website www.gotpaindocs.com under occipital neuralgia or YouTube.com in the channel for drjohnpetraglia or painmangementbeyond or thepaindoctors

Diagnosis and Treatment

There is no specific test for migraine headaches. It is worth noting that several diseases and conditions may mimic migraines, such as glaucoma, sinusitis, and brain abnormalities such as blood clots, brain tumors, and abscesses. All patients with a history of migraines undergoing a change in symptoms, or those with new symptoms, should undergo magnetic resonance imaging (MRI) of the brain. Eye examination should be pursued in those patients who have persistent ocular symptoms.

In making the decision with your physician on how best to treat migraines, one should consider the following: the frequency and severity of headaches, the effect on lifestyle, the presence or absence of prolonged neurological disturbances, the history of drug use, and the presence of other diseases that may rule out certain treatment options. In general, if the migraines occur infrequently, then *abortive therapy* is probably a better option. If the headaches occur often, interfere with daily life, and result in trips to the emergency room, then *prophylactic therapy* is recommended.

For abortive therapy to work, it generally must be started at the first sign of headache. Medications commonly used to stop migraines include nonsteroidal anti-inflammatory drugs such as Ibuprofen and Naprosyn. It has also been reported that the inhalation of pure oxygen may stop migraine headaches before they progress. Other classes of medication that may treat migraine headaches contain caffeine, barbiturates, ergot, and triptans. As a word of caution, medications that contain caffeine, barbiturates, ergot preparations, amines, and triptans may contribute to an analgesic rebound headache, which occurs when the medication taken initially to abort the migraine wears off.

Prophylactic therapy is advisable for people who suffer from migraine headaches that regularly interrupt their daily lives. This consists of using drugs known as *beta-blocking agents*. The most famous drug of this type is Propanolol, which decreases the frequency and intensity of migraine headaches and helps prevent aura.

More recently, BOTOX has been used and is now FDA approved to treat migraines with moderate success. Yes, the very same BOTOX that is used to treat wrinkles can also block the vasodilating effect of proteins that act on the vessels of the brain. In other words, theory holds that the BOTOX effect may increase blood flow to critical areas of the brain, relaxing tension areas involved in precipitating a full-blown migraine. Many insurance carriers are slow to acknowledge the benefit of BOTOX in reducing migraines. The insurance companies are concerned because it will be costly to offer BOTOX therapy to them, this may then create a surge of requests for BOTOX treatment. However, clinical studies have proven a decrease in intensity and severity of migraine headaches with its use. Currently the recommendation is to provide chronic migraine sufferers H/A fifteen times per month with at least 150 units of BOTOX injected into a specific muscle group in the face and neck.

Finally, it is important to remember that if a migraine headache does not respond to traditional treatments such as BOTOX or Triptan medication, the headache may actually be of a different type.

Case Study: *I have treated many migraine patients with BOTOX. In my experience, if a headache does not respond to BOTOX treatment it is, more than likely, another type of headache. I'm reminded of Suzanne, a woman who went to great lengths to treat her headaches. Different pain management doctors performed various procedures to try to diminish her pain. Many medication regimens were tried, most of which made her sick to her stomach. When I met her, I suggested a BOTOX injection. This worked amazingly well, and now she gets a booster BOTOX injection for headaches every six months to keep her headaches under control. She takes very little other medication and is able to keep her chronic migraine headaches to a minimum using this therapy.*

Tension Type Headaches

A tension type headache is even more common than a migraine. Often, people who suffer from tension type headaches experience significant sleep disturbances and depression. The depression can often spiral into a serious condition impacting their work and relationships. These headaches typically involve the frontal and temporal sides of the head, as well as the back of the scalp.

The headache comes on as a series of nonpulsing, band-like aches experienced as "tightness in the scalp." This is usually accompanied by neck tenderness. Tension type headaches can last hours or even days and remain constant. Tension headaches usually occur between 4:00 a.m. and 8:00 a.m., and between 4:00 p.m. and 8:00 p.m. As with migraines, females tend to suffer from this type of headache more frequently than males. The timing of the headache may correlate to the fluctuating levels of cortisol and neuro transmitters, essential chemicals in the body.

Tension type headaches are typically triggered by physical or psychological stress. For example, driving for long hours, craning the neck, or dealing with a particularly heavy workload at work may precipitate this type of headache.

Diagnosis and Treatment

As with migraines, there is no specific test for tension type headaches. An MRI should be performed on the brain, and if the pain is in the back or near the neck, the cervical spine should be scanned as well.

Tension type headaches are often confused with migraines, but they can be distinguished in a number of ways. First of all, migraine headaches have a minute to one hour onset-to-peak duration. In tension type headaches, this onset-to-peak intensity may take hours to days. Migraines rarely occur more than once a week, while tension type headaches may occur daily. Migraines are typically located on the side of the scalp, while tension type headaches are in the back of the neck or around the head. Migraines tend to consist of pounding pain, while tension type headaches involve aching with a band-like pressure. Unlike migraines, tension type headaches usually affect both sides of the head, and there is no aura during the onset. Also, with tension type headaches nausea and vomiting are rare. Nausea and vomiting are more common with migraine headaches.

Analgesics and nonsteroidal anti-inflammatory drugs are commonly used to treat tension type headaches. Antidepressants normalize sleep patterns of the sufferers, treat their depression, and may be effective in decreasing the frequency and intensity of these headaches. Doctors may also prescribe drugs like Amitriptyline, Trazodone, and Fluoxetine as part of the treatment.

Many studies have shown the effectiveness of cervical epidural nerve blocks in providing long-term relief of tension type headaches. Such cervical epidural steroid injections may be performed daily to weekly as necessary to control symptoms. If depression is a significant component of the tension headaches, in my experience it proves beneficial to treat depression first before the headache is aggravated. There are a multitude of good antidepressant medications, which generally work by blocking the reuptake of certain brain chemicals known as neurotransmitters.

Acute Herpes Zoster Headaches

Herpes zoster is an infectious disease similar to chickenpox. Headaches stemming from this condition may occur when the herpes zoster virus attacks the geniculate ganglion (in the hand) resulting in pain, vesicle formation in the ear, and hearing loss.

Treatment

Treatments include sympathetic nerve blocks with local anesthetics and steroids. Sympathetic nerve blocks are not injections performed in sympathy. They are an injection at certain nerve sites in the sympathetic nerve system. Sympathetic nerve blocks are directed toward the *stellate ganglion* located in the neck and the *trigeminal ganglion*, located in the face. Opioid analgesics, anticonvulsants, and antiviral agents can be used in conjunction with nerve blocks to provide relief in most patients. The application of ice will also dull the pain in most patients.

Cluster Headaches

As the name suggests, these headaches come in clusters. Males are five times more likely to suffer from them than females, and roughly 0.5 percent of the US male population experiences them. They are less common than migraines or tension type headaches and normally affect patients in their thirties and forties, as opposed to migraines, which can begin manifesting themselves in patients in their early twenties or even earlier.

The cluster headache usually starts ninety minutes after the patient falls asleep. It also appears to follow a biological pattern that coincides with seasonal changes and the length of days. Consequently, cluster headaches happen more frequently in the spring and fall.

During a cluster event, headaches occur two or three times a day lasting forty-five minutes to an hour. The cluster event itself will usually last for eight to twelve weeks, with usually a minimum of two years between events. However, in patients with chronic cluster headache, the frequency of the cluster events steadily increases.

Like the migraine, a cluster headache usually happens on one side of the head, behind the eye. The pain consists of a deep burning or boring quality and is often extreme and intense. The pain has been likened to having your eye or the top of your head penetrated. Several female patients have said it is worse than the pain of giving birth. Other symptoms include drooping eyelids, abnormal pupil constriction, redness of the eyes, facial flushing, excess tearing and/or a runny nose. The headache can be triggered by small amounts of alcohol, nitrates, histamines, and occasionally by high altitudes.

Though these headaches are rare, they are quite serious. Patients suffering from chronic cluster headaches that are difficult to manage can experience severe depression, with unrelenting pain, and have been known to commit suicide.

Diagnosis and Treatment

As with other headache syndromes, MRI studies should be performed on the brain and/or neck region. Treatment of cluster headaches may involve oral steroid medication combined with the application of *sphenopalatine ganglion* blocks with a local anesthetic. The sphenopalatine ganglion is a collection of nerve cell bodies deep behind the nose region. An anesthetization of these cells will diminish the symptoms. Also, inhalation of pure oxygen may be used as a preventative measure. Other common medications used to treat this type of headache include lithium carbonate, methysergide, and sumatriptan.

Medication (Analgesic) Rebound Headache

Recently identified, this syndrome afflicts headache sufferers who overuse abortive medications to treat their migraines or tension type headaches. Since a migraine or a tension type headache can transform into an analgesic rebound headache, the latter will have characteristics of both. The common trigger medications include simple analgesics such as sinus medications, aspirin, caffeine, and butalbitals such as Fiorinal. However, overusing nonsteroidal anti-inflammatory drugs, opioid analgesics, and the triptans may also spur the headache on. Precisely because of overmedication, analgesic rebound headaches become unresponsive to abortive and prophylactic medications.

Diagnosis and Treatment

All patients should undergo MRI studies of the brain and neck region. Treatment of the analgesic rebound headache involves first and foremost the discontinuation of the overused medication for a period of at least three months. Unfortunately, the headache symptoms may get worse before they get better.

Occipital Neuralgia

Occipital neuralgia is usually the result of trauma to the occipital nerves. Repetitive hyperextension of the neck (such as working with computer monitors that are at an elevated level) may precipitate this condition. The pain is persistent and is located at the base of the skull. It comes in the form of sudden, shock-like, sharp nerve impulses. The condition may also be brought on by trauma to the head or neck such as suffered in a car accident. A whiplash injury may give rise to occipital neuralgia at the site of the nerve at the base of the scalp.

Diagnosis and Treatment

Occipital nerve blocks, namely injections of a local anesthetic with a steroid, will treat occipital neuralgia very well. Sometimes, tension type headaches can mimic the behavior of occipital neuralgia. However, if the headaches are of tension type, they will not respond to occipital nerve blocks. They are treated with antidepressant medication and cervical epidural steroid injections. Thus, an injection of occipital nerve blocks may serve to diagnostically prove or disprove the existence of occipital neuralgia. Please see website Gotpaindocs.com video archive of occipital nerve block or visit youtube.com "drjohnpetraglia" or "the pain doctors."

Case Study *Lisa told me about headaches she's been having since childhood. They were severe enough to significantly impact her ability to work. She took a series of pills on different days to stop, or at least diminish, her pain.*

I examined Lisa carefully and saw that there appeared to be two different subgroups of headaches. One had a vascular component that triggered a migraine, which incapacitated the patient and interfered with her work. The other consisted of continuous throbbing and a heavy sensation suggestive of occipital neuralgia.

Lisa entered the office with dark glasses and a hat, concealing almost her entire head, protecting her from the light she found so painful. We conducted our interview in a semilit room without windows, an eerie setting for a patient-doctor conversation. She had walked in the office angry and miserable, almost in tears because of the excruciating headache pain. After our consultation, we agreed to perform an occipital nerve block. Within ten minutes of the procedure her headache disappeared.

Amazed at the simplicity of the solution to a problem she found so unbearable, Lisa was elated beyond words. I still see her occasionally for follow-ups but she has never experienced headaches of that magnitude again.

Headache Questionnaire–Answer these questions to map pain symptoms

*(Copy and fill out these worksheets and bring to your doctor. He/she may have his/her own worksheets, but answers to these questions provide a good overview of your pain condition and will help you remember and gather a full **pain profile** in order to use your time with your doctor more effectively.)*

Where is your pain located?

When does your pain start and end?

When did you first begin to have pain, to the best of your recollection?

Where does your pain travel to?

Is it continuous throughout the day?

Has your pain ever improved?

Has it become chronic?

Are there two or more different types of pain syndromes that seem to occur simultaneously?

Does your pain wax and wane, or does it stay at the same intensity throughout the course of the day?

Does the pain occur all over?

Which pain bothers you the most?

Do the different pains that you have come from different areas and appear to be related to different conditions or movements of the face or body?

Which pain would you like to get rid of the most?

Do you have a systemic disease diagnosed previously that may be contributing to your pain?

Do you believe your pain is caused by accident or injury?

Was this a work-related injury?

Could an old injury that did not heal be exacerbated by current daily activities?

Use the following scale to describe the severity of your pain for each type of pain you have,

with 1 being the least amount of pain and 10 being the highest level of pain you could ever imagine: 1 … 2 … 3 … 4 … 5 … 6 … 7 … 8 … 9 … 10.

What descriptors can you use for your pain: Burning? Aching? Shooting? Sharp? Throbbing? Cramping? Constant? Numbing? Lancinating? Stabbing? Transient? Excruciating? Tingling? On fire?

Does your pain get worse or better with sitting, bending, lifting, walking, grasping, sweeping, standing, crawling, squatting, reaching overhead, eating, coughing, sneezing, physical activity, stress, driving, sexual intercourse, heat, ice, physical therapy, medications?

Have any of the following treatments provided relief of your pain condition: Surgery? Medications? Injection therapy? Chiropractic? Tens unit (electric stimulation)? Physical therapy? Traction? Heat therapy? Rest? Acupuncture? Psychotherapy?

Does the pain seem to arise in the head or neck, or does it appear to come from another area that can be directed to the top of the head? _____ Side of the head? Directly behind the eyeball? _____ Shoot from the back to the front in a ram's horn type of distribution? _____

Is the headache pain fleeting, transient, intermittent, or does it come in waves or cycles? Is the pain constant and/or throbbing? _____ Is the pain sharp? Is the headache pain associated with a vascular phenomenon? _____ menstrual periods? _____ premenstrual syndrome? _____

If you have had extensive dental work, do you still have pain coming from the teeth? _____ Does this appear to cause or to contribute to headaches? _____ Have you had extensive dental extractions? _____ Root canals? _____

Have you had extensive silver fillings or dental implants? _____

Is the headache pain associated with: Numbness or tingling _____ Weakness of any of the muscles of the face or scalp? _____ Paralysis? _____ Increased or decreased sweating? _____ Skin discoloration? _____ Skin rash anywhere on the face or head? _____Tingling pins and needles on the face or body? _____ Cold? _____ Muscle spasm tightness? _____ Trouble sleeping? _____ "Touch me not" pain? _____

Is there a history of oral or facial herpes? _____

What improves your headache pain? _____ What medications have you tried that have failed? _____ Have you had injections for your headache pain?

_____ Occipital nerve block? BOTOX? _____ Other type of facial or head injection? _____

What specifically helps your headaches: Sleep? _____ Rest? _____ Ice? _____ Heat? _____Pressure? Exercise? _____ Any type of therapy? _____ Any kind of surgery? _____ Have you used light or laser therapy to try to treat your headache pain? _____

What specific medications have you tried or failed? _____

What specific herbal or natural remedies have you tried? _____

Do you take supplements for your condition? _____

Do you get rebound headaches after taking medicine for headaches? _____ Is your pain accompanied with headaches? _____ How would you best describe these headaches? _____

Is your pain accompanied with temporary paralysis? _____ Do the muscles of your face or head go into spasm or become distorted at any time? _____ Do the expressions of the facial muscles or scalp appear to be weaker at any time? _____

Body map for headache pain questionnaire

Please refer to the website www.gotpaindocs.com, www.thegreatPainJack.com, or www. thegreatPainJack.org, for further information.

Figure 1B

Occipital View

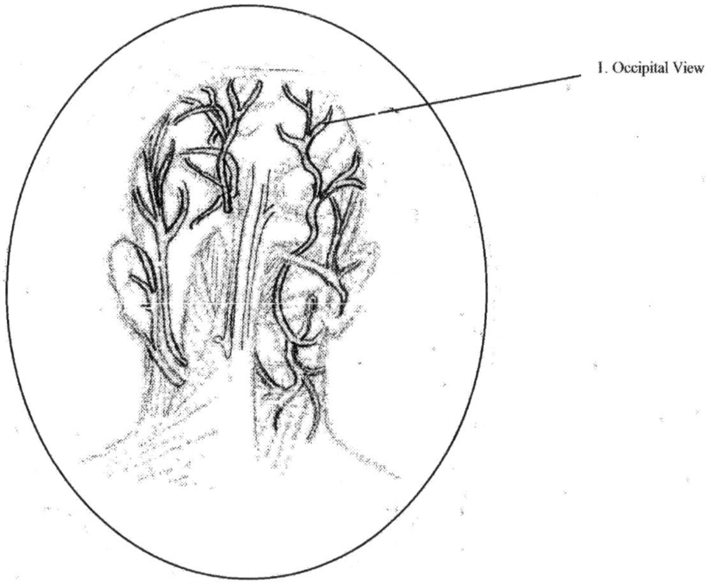

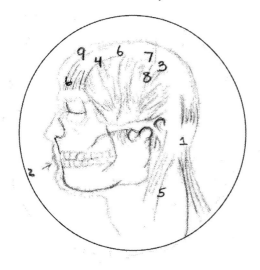

1. Occipital View

Figure 1A

Headache Pain Syndromes

1. Occipital Neuralgia
2. Analgesic Rebound Headache
3. Tension-Type Headache
4. Migraine Headache
5. Herpes Zoster 1st Division of the Trigeminal Nerve
6. Cluster Headache
7. Ice Pick Headache
8. Chronic Paroxysmal Hemicrania
9. Post-Dural Puncture Headache

Figure 2

Occipital Neuralgia

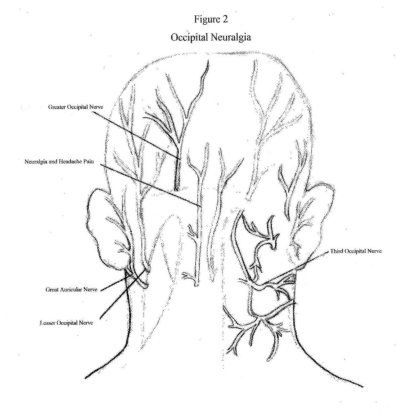

Greater Occipital Nerve

Neuralgia and Headache Pain

Third Occipital Nerve

Great Auricular Nerve

Lesser Occipital Nerve

Figure 3

Headache Pain Syndrome

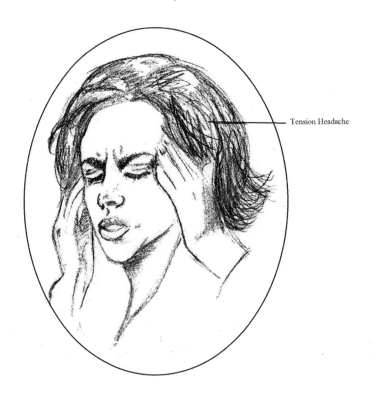

Tension Headache

Chapter 6

So You've Got Facial Pain?

Case Study: Mary, a young mother of five, has had facial pain and jaw asymmetry most of her life. The jaw asymmetry has led to a facial grimace that has worn at the jaw joint prematurely. She undergoes regular injection therapy to minimize the symptoms, allowing her to function and completely cut down on medication with very little maintenance.

A facial pain syndrome can be one of the most severe and debilitating conditions to experience. I have seen and treated countless types of severe and intractable facial afflictions that would not heal on their own. Here, I address trigeminal neuralgia, temporomandibular joint dysfunction, atypical facial pain, and reflex sympathetic dystrophy of the face. However, this is a mere sampling of the conditions that can ultimately cause facial pain.

Trigeminal Neuralgia

Trigeminal neuralgia (TN) causes pain so incredibly intense that it has been nicknamed "the suicide disease." It affects the trigeminal nerves, which travel through the face. The pain is characterized by intense electric shocks lasting a few seconds to a few minutes. Activities such as brushing the teeth, washing the face, or shaving the skin may lead to neuralgic attacks. Between TN attacks, the pain of trigeminal neuralgia is relatively small. A dull ache can sometimes remain after the intense shock-like pain dissipates. The condition is occasionally associated with multiple sclerosis. Patients with coexisting multiple sclerosis may have other symptoms, such as dementia and weakness.

Diagnosis and Treatment

Diagnostic testing should include MRI evaluation of the brain and brain stem. Magnetic resonance angiography can be used to check vein compression in the trigeminal nerves. Also, an ophthalmologist eye exam should be carried out to measure pressure inside both eyes. Elevated intraocular pressure may be an ominous sign.

Case Study: *Rene, a young nurse, experienced sharp pain, which she felt above the eye. This condition had been going on for some time and was not responding to medication therapy. Other attempts to treat her, like surgical microvascular decompression of the fifth nerve, gamma knife ablation of the gasserian ganglion, and neurostimulator trials all failed, and the last procedure made her pain significantly worse. Her family physician was running out of options and decided to refer her to me.*

As a nurse, she was unable to take pain medications that would ultimately affect her ability to perform her job. Thus, during her treatments she was forced to go on disability. As a result, she soon lost her health insurance and job, and, with it, hope for relief.

Generally with surgical procedures the potential for additional side effects and complications of the surgery and additionally painful scar tissue formation all become a possible outcome scenario. I believe that is what ultimately affected Rene and caused her condition to deteriorate. The increasingly large quantities of medication she needed to take daily eventually led to her inability to perform her job as a nurse. Unable to perform her job, she became depressed and lost her income. In pain management, we don't always have happy endings.

Case Study: *Jim, a young educator, once complained to me of facial pain after having dental work done. He said his pain was sharp and felt "electrically charged" in his face. He learned that he had developed a chronic pain condition involving the trigeminal nerve. It had been investigated extensively with an MRI, exploratory surgery attempting to rejoin severed nerves, x-rays, and brain scans. He had been to a number of practitioners that either refused to treat him or did not know how to diagnose his condition.*

After a careful diagnosis, I attempted to provide several treatments, including deep brain stimulation, magnetic and injection therapy, and various medications, which he found difficult to tolerate. We further agreed on a combination of injections involving botulism type A toxin for muscular pain and injections into the nerve cells of the trigeminal nerve, deep within the face. In the course of three years, Jim had at least twelve facial injections. Though painful, these injections alleviated his condition tremendously.

A first-line treatment medication is *carbamazepine.* The response to this drug can confirm a diagnosis of trigeminal neuralgia. However, carbamazepine can cause significant abnormalities, like rashes and blood irregularities, which necessitate a complete blood count, serum chemistry, and urine analysis prior to prescription. Carbamazepine therapy should be started slowly with increasing dosage.

Neurontin is an antiseizure medication that can also be used to treat TN. Neurontin, like carbamazepine, unfortunately comes with its share of side effects, which include dizziness, confusion, and rashes. *Baclofen*, an antispasm medication, has been helpful in reducing some of the lancinating pain that TN triggers. Sudden withdrawal from any of these medications may cause the pain to return and make it less manageable in the future.

A trigeminal nerve block with a local anesthetic steroid can also provide relief. These nerve blocks should be injected as necessary to control pain. Equally, the injection of glycerol into the convergence of the nerve cells in the trigeminal nerve, known as the gasserian ganglion, can provide long-term relief for patients with TN. The destruction of the gasserian ganglion is performed on patients who have been healed by other treatments.

Temporomandibular Joint Dysfunction

Temporomandibular joint dysfunction (TMD) affects the temporomandibular joint, which connects the jaw to the skull. We use this joint on a daily basis, for example when eating, thus the condition can be very debilitating. The pain stemming from this condition radiates into the jaw, ear, tonsils, and neck. TMD can be caused by stress or dental malalignment, but also by a traumatic event such as a car accident. The patient may experience increasing pain and limitation of jaw movement, as well as headaches. If arthritis is present in the joint, opening and closing may result in clicking or grating. Primarily, however, TMD gives rise to debilitating neck pain.

Case Study: I once examined a pleasant, heavyset woman, Bethann, who complained of headaches and neck pain from a car accident twelve years prior. She had been taking significant doses of narcotics ever since, and, despite being well-adjusted to the medication intake, Bethann missed as many as three to five days of work a week due to the pain.

After the exam, Bethann told me that she felt moderate relief after cervical facet injections performed by a previous doctor. Since she hadn't had a cervical MRI or a neck x-ray in a while, I recommended both. There were minimal findings on the MRI in the form of cervical disc herniations.

As Bethann related the type and character of her pain, I began to realize that she was attaching a huge emotional component to the accident, possibly magnifying the actual physical pain she felt. I explored this theory by performing a cervical epidural steroid injection with an occipital nerve block to treat the cervical disc herniations and headaches. And so, after twelve years, she finally experienced relief and stopped taking the rather large dose of her regular pain medications.

After a while, however, her pain slowly returned. During the follow-up visit I reexamined her head and neck more thoroughly. During the exam, I discovered a significant clicking and major displacement of the jaw. I ordered an MRI of her jaw, and the results were astonishing. The meniscus within her temporomandibular joint was almost entirely dislocated, and there was an abnormal accumulation of fluid within the joint. When she opened and closed her mouth she exerted pressure on the main muscle on the side of the face known as the maseter. This action reproduced her headaches.

When I explained the situation to her and her fiancé, both seemed at peace with the diagnosis, gaining an insight into her condition. We discussed surgical options, as well as temporomandibular joint steroid injections, which at the time of writing of this book are still on the table as a treatment option.

Diagnosis and Treatment

TMD requires evaluation to rule out infectious and inflammatory causes, including collagen vascular diseases. When temporomandibular joint pain occurs in older patients, the pain should be differentiated from jaw pain associated with the inflammation of the arteries of the side of the face. MRI studies of the temporomandibular joint can help identify any abnormalities in the joint. Dental and sinus problems, reflex sympathetic dystrophy of the face and atypical facial pain can also be mistaken for TMD. Finally, tumors of the jawbone and pharynx can produce TMJ pain and should be evaluated by your physician.

Treatment of TMJ can involve oral orthotic devices and physical therapy as well as injection of small amounts of local anesthetic and steroid. Antidepressant medications can also improve the underlying pain. A night guard can prevent problems caused by jaw clenching and grinding of the teeth, both of which can exacerbate TMD. Surgical treatment to restore normal joint function is very rare.

Case Study: So Hin, a young Korean woman who spoke little English, was involved in a car accident, and she complained to her doctors of severe jaw pain. She claimed she was unable to eat, and anything that touched her face caused her immense pain. Since the car accident was rather minor, coupled with the fact that her spoken English was poor, doctors tended to believe she was gravely exaggerating.

Yet, for six months she could not even open her mouth and chew her food. She lost weight and became irritable, and her family life was continuously disrupted. When I saw her, I recommended an MRI of her jaw, which revealed a dislocated meniscus of the temporomandibular joint. I treated her with a series of injections in the jaw, which healed her pain. Soon she could eat and live a normal life.

Atypical Facial Pain

Atypical facial pain, also known as atypical facial neuralgia, is a term used to describe a group of syndromes causing facial pain. A main precipitating factor of atypical facial pain is stress. Also, a prior history of facial trauma, infection, or tumors may play a triggering role. However, in certain patients no triggers have been found.

Patients diagnosed with this condition tend to be female. The pain is often continuous and varies in intensity. It is almost always one-sided and consists of aching or cramping rather than shock-like, lancinating, or neuritic pain typical of trigeminal neuralgia. It is like a constant dull ache. Headaches resembling tension types frequently accompany atypical facial pain. Difficulty sleeping and depression are common in patients who suffer from this disorder.

> **Case Study:** *Jerome, a middle-aged man, was referred to me by his neurologist. The neurologist said that he had problems diagnosing and treating the man's eight-month history of left-sided atypical facial pain. MRI studies and CAT scans were all benign. To complicate things, Jerome had a strange eruption of a tooth that occurred fifteen years after his wisdom teeth were pulled. Jerome described a strange sensation of roughness along the gum line, on the side of the mouth closest to the tongue. He also felt numbness in a part of his tongue, on the left side. Strangely, his neck swelled and felt sore on that side.*
>
> *These symptoms could point to a variety of conditions. I incorporated the diagnostic acumen of an ear, nose, and throat specialist as well as a fantastic neurologist to help determine the cause of Jerome's condition. We suspect that the regrowth of tooth material may be responsible for his pain, but we do not have a definite answer yet. Going off our current atypical facial pain diagnosis, Jerome will receive a series of facial and trigeminal blocks until we can determine a more specific cause.*
>
> *His workup included evaluation for the possibility of the eagle's syndrome, an abnormal condition whereby an elongated bone known as the styloid process may poke a vital structure such as a branch of nerve or nerve center in the lower jaw and neck area. X-ray studies did not prove this. ENT larngoscopy failed to reveal any sign of a tumor or explanation for the condition.*
>
> *As of the writing of this book, Jerome has undergone a series of behavioral cognitive retraining sessions with our pain psychologist. His condition was complicated by the development of small stroke or brain infarct, which occurred in the movement balance central areas of the brain. To date the neurologist has been unable to classify the quirky, jerky movement disorder he has subsequently developed.*

Diagnosis and Treatment

X-rays of the head as well as MRI imaging of the brain and sinuses will help differentiate pathology within the brain. If inflammatory arthritis or temporal arteritis is suspected, blood tests or a biopsy may be performed to confirm the diagnosis.

Generally, atypical facial pain is diagnosed by excluding other possible causes for pain. Infection and inflammatory causes, and temporal arthritis (in older patients) should be investigated first. One way to tell atypical facial pain apart from trigeminal neuralgia is that patients with the former will often rub affected areas, while people with TN will avoid rubbing their faces at all costs. The clinical signs of atypical facial pain may also be confused with pain due to dental or sinus problems.

In terms of treatment, atypical facial pain does not respond to the ganglion blocks mentioned earlier. Instead, a combination of antidepressant therapy, orthotic devices, and physical therapy should be prescribed. Injections of anesthetics and steroids into both the trigeminal nerve and the temporomandibular may also relieve the pain.

Reflex Sympathetic Dystrophy

The common denominator in patients suffering from reflex sympathetic dystrophy of the face, or RSD, is tissue trauma. This may take the form of injury to the soft tissue or the teeth or bones of the face, infection and cancer, or arthritis and damage to the central nervous system or cranial nerves. The hallmark of RSD is a burning pain, often located in the skin, or painful sensations that are associated with stimuli that actually produces the pain. Trigger areas are especially common inside the mouth. Subtle skin color changes as well as odd changes in blood flow of facial skin may accompany RSD. Patients suffering from it may have had dental extractions that were performed as pain-reducing procedures. The condition typically results in depression and sleep problems.

Diagnosis and Treatment

A presumptive diagnosis of RSD can be made if the patient gets adequate relief after a stellate ganglion block. Other potential causes of pain, including tumors, temporal arthritis, or collagen vascular disease should first be excluded. The clinical signs of RSD of the face can also be confused with dental and sinus diseases, as well as atypical facial pain. MRI imaging of the brain and cervical spine should also be carried out to make a thorough diagnosis. RSD should be suspected in any patient who has pain associated with preexisting trauma or pain that is burning.

Treatment involves eliminating the cause of tissue trauma contributing to the condition. RSD patients respond well to sympathetic nerve blocks at the stellate ganglion. Antidepressants and sleep medication should be used to treat the depression and sleep disorders associated with this condition. Drugs such as Lyrica and/or Neurontin may help diminish the neuritic or neuropathic pain. Regular blockade of the sympathetic nerves in the pain areas will confirm the diagnosis and reduce symptoms.

Please refer to the website www.gotpaindocs.com, www.thegreatPainJack.com, or www.thegreatPainJack.org, for further information.

Herpes

Occasionally herpes virus or an attack of "shingles" can attack the nerves of the face. This can lead to loss of vision and the development of an extremely painful condition. The condition should be treated early.

> ***Case Study:*** *Arun, an elderly woman, came to my office with a terrible rash above her eye, discoloration of the skin, and an anguishing, irritating pain. At first glance, this appeared to be a herpes attack of the first division of the fifth cranial nerve. She came to our clinic and received the medication she needed to diminish the symptoms and duration of the shingles attack on her face.*
>
> *Since her regular clinic was in a rural, agricultural area surrounded by mountains and fairly isolated, without easy medical access, I was glad that she had been treated by our office. Since we diagnosed her condition early, we were able to start treating it in its early stages and heal it completely.*

Conditions involving shingles of any of the divisions of the trigeminal nerve that involve the face can be difficult to treat in the later stages of development. Therefore, prompt diagnosis and treatment are keys to healing the condition.

Facial Pain Questionnaire–Answer these questions to map pain symptoms

*(Copy and fill out these worksheets and bring to your doctor. He/she may have his/her own, but answers to these questions provide a good overview of your pain condition and will help you remember and collect a **pain profile** in order to use your time with your doctor more effectively.)*

Where is your pain located? _____

When does your pain start and end? _____

When did you first begin to have pain, to the best of your recollection? _____
_____

Where does your pain travel to? _____

Is it continuous throughout the day? _____

Has your pain ever improved? _____

Has it become chronic? _____

Are there two or more different types of pain syndromes that seem to occur simultaneously?
_____

Does your pain wax and wane, or does it stay at the same intensity throughout the course of the day? _____

Does the pain occur all over? _____

Which pain bothers you the most? _____

Do the different pains that you have come from different areas and appear to be related to different conditions or movements of the face or body? _____

Which pain would you like to get rid of the most? _____

Do you have a systemic disease diagnosed previously that may be contributing to your pain? _____

Do you believe your pain is caused by accident or injury? _____

Was this a work-related injury? _____

Could an old injury that did not heal be exacerbated by current daily activities? _____
_____

Use the following scale to describe the severity of your pain for each type of pain you have with one being the least amount of pain and 10 being the highest level of pain you could ever imagine: 1 ... 2 ... 3 ... 4 ... 5 ... 6 ... 7 ... 8 ... 9 ... 10.

What descriptors can you use for your pain: Burning? Aching? Shooting? Sharp? Throbbing? Cramping? Constant? Numbing? Lancinating? Stabbing? Transient? Excruciating? Tingling? On fire? Other?

Does your pain get worse or better with sitting, bending, lifting, walking, grasping, sweeping, standing, crawling, squatting, reaching overhead, eating, coughing, sneezing, physical activity, stress, driving, sexual intercourse, heat, ice, physical therapy, medications?

Have any of the following treatments provided relief of your pain condition: Surgery? Medications? Injection therapy? Chiropractic? Tens unit (electric stimulation)? Physical therapy? Traction? Heat therapy? Bed rest? Acupuncture? Psychotherapy?

Specific questions regarding facial pain to best allow you and your doctor to make a diagnosis

Does the pain seem to arise in the face or does it appear to come from another area that can be directed to the face? _____

Is the facial pain fleeting, transient, or constant and throbbing? _____

If you have had extensive dental work, do you still have pain coming from the teeth? _____ Have you had extensive dental extractions? _____

Is the facial pain associated with: Numbness? _____ Weakness? _____ Paralysis? _____ Increased or decreased sweating? _____ Skin discoloration? _____ Skin rash anywhere on the face or body? _____ Tingling pins and needles on the face or body? _____ Cold? _____ Muscle spasm tightness? _____ Trouble sleeping? _____ "Touch me not" pain? _____

What improves your facial pain? _____ What medications have you tried that failed? _____ Have you had injections for your pain?

What specifically helps your facial pain: Sleep? _____ Rest? _____ Ice? _____ Heat? _____ Pressure? _____ Exercise? _____ Any type of therapy? _____ Any kind of surgery? _____ Have you used light or laser therapy to try to treat your facial pain?

What specific medications have you tried? _____

What specific herbal or natural remedies have you tried? _____

Do you take supplements for your condition? _____

Is your pain accompanied with headaches? _____

How would you best describe these headaches? _____

Is your pain accompanied with transient paralysis? _____ Do the muscles of your face go into spasm or become distorted at any time? _____

Do the expressions of the facial muscles appear to be weaker at any time? _____

Body Map for Facial Pain Questionnaire

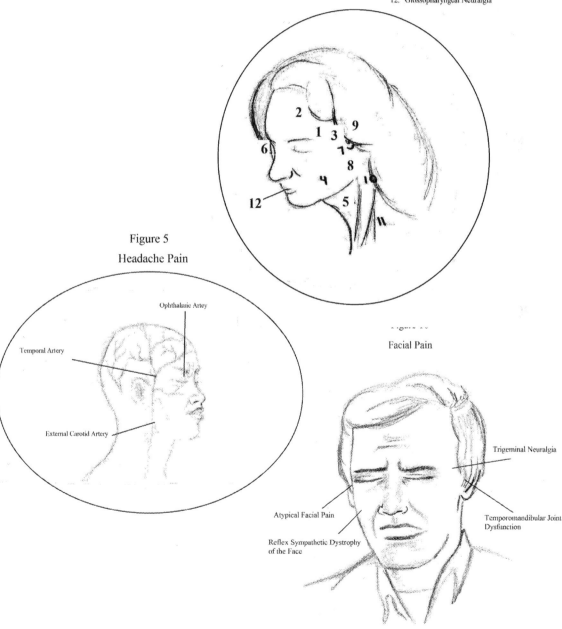

Figure 4
Facial Pain

1. Migraine Headache
2. Herpes Zoster of the 1st Division
3. Trigeminal Neuralgia
4. Reflex Sympathetic Dystrophy of the Face
5. Cancer of the Face, Neck or Body
6. Temporomandibular Joint Dysfunction
7. Atypical Facial Pain
8. RSD of the Face
9. Ramsay Hunt Syndrome
10. Eagle's Syndrome
11. Omohyoid Syndrome
12. Glossopharyngeal Neuralgia

Figure 5

Headache Pain

Ophthalmic Artey

Temporal Artery

External Carotid Artery

Facial Pain

Trigeminal Neuralgia

Atypical Facial Pain

Temporomandibular Joint Dysfunction

Reflex Sympathetic Dystrophy of the Face

Chapter 7:

So, You've Got Abdominal Pain?

Case Study: *I was covering as a staff anesthesiologist early one Sunday morning at a local hospital. The shift had been very routine, so I decided to go get some breakfast on site. As I finished my breakfast and headed to the parking lot I heard a 911 page calling for me. Apparently there was a man with a ruptured abdominal aortic aneurysm in the emergency room that needed urgent attention.*

*T*his was a pure and simple life-or-death situation. I ran to the emergency department, only to find that the patient was already taken to the x-ray suite. The patient, a sixty-three-year-old male, was exiting the CAT scan machine, screaming in agony.

The cardiothoracic surgeon's eyes caught mine. He was holding the CAT scan results. I swallowed hard. We examined them silently. The full meaning of what we were looking at slowly sunk in. The surgeon cursed under his breath. Again and again.

The old man's cries continued, undiminished. His aorta, the body's main arterial supply, was literally disintegrating into his abdomen. Without medical intervention he would die soon.

We had to act fast. The surgeon and I ran the gurney up the elevator and rushed the man into the operating room. I rapidly instructed the nursing staff to type and cross units of blood, fresh frozen plasma, platelets, and any other type of fluid we could pump into this man to sustain his life vital fluids. The surgeon opened the chest, perhaps before I was able to get a breathing tube down his trachea. Blood gushed everywhere. I called for backup and had two nurses pump fluid and blood through large intravenous catheters placed in his arms and neck.

I wanted to place a special arterial line catheter to track the patient's blood pressure, but it was difficult to find an artery that had an arterial pulse in his wrist for such measurement. Miraculously, the arterial line somehow found its way into the right vessel, and I breathed a sigh of relief. My relief was short-lived as I realized that the blood pressure was so low, it was difficult to measure.

As the surgeon reconstructed what was left of the man's aorta, patching it with a Gortex graft, we pumped blood, plasma, and platelets into his body. Though I couldn't get a solid *blood pressure reading for what must have been now an hour and a half, we still had a heart rate. This gave us hope.*

The cardiothoracic surgeon muttered: "This patient should have never been taken to this hospital. The last three patients I've had here with this condition have all died on the table!" But I was determined to not allow the man's life to end this way. Maybe it was my father's spirit of perseverance awakening inside me: "I would not, could not, quit." Though it's a cliché, I've learned over the years that it holds a lot of truth. I would not let this man die on my watch. It was as simple as that.

The intense struggle to save the patient lasted approximately two hours. We were all exhausted now. We transported the patient to ICU for postoperative monitoring. I asked for ventilator management, critical care monitoring with measurement of arterial blood gases, blood oxygen saturation, and minute-by-minute blood pressure and pulse measurement.

Five hours had passed. Drinking an umpteenth cup of coffee, I was approached by a nurse. She informed me that the patient had woken up, pulled out his breathing tube, and asked for food. I could not believe my ears. Five hours after nearly dying, with barely any blood pressure, the man wanted his dinner!

I drank my coffee, thinking only about sleep.

The workup for abdominal pain can be very extensive. There are a great many possible conditions that can give rise to pain in the abdomen. Some of the most familiar include gastrointestinal tract disorders like hernias or ulcers, Crohn's disease, appendicitis, endometriosis, painful ovulation, cancer, ulcerative colitis, gallbladder disease, twisting or rotation of the bowel, abdominal parasites such as worms, and bacterial infection. Acute abdominal pain from conditions such as appendicitis, acute bowel obstruction, or the rupture of an aneurysm frequently require surgical intervention.

Chronic abdominal pain, on the other hand, rarely results in surgery. A diagnosis evaluating chronic abdominal pain would include a CAT scan or an endoscopy, which consists of putting a camera inside the stomach or inside the upper and lower gastrointestinal tract. Barium or radio-opaque IV contrast dye studies and laparoscopic evaluation may also be employed to make a diagnosis. Stool examination should be performed to determine the presence of a parasite living in the colon or the GI tract. This procedure is highly recommended for people with abdominal discomfort who travel a lot, particularly to countries with contaminated water or food.

Case Study: *Joelle, a very successful businesswoman, came to see me, concerned about possible hormone dysfunction, chronic diarrhea, and weight loss. She'd been to many doctors, yet nothing was detected during a routine endoscopy, an examination of the gastrointestinal tract.*

When I met her she was very thin and said she felt immense fatigue all day long. She complained of chronic diarrhea, which she attributed to irritable bowel syndrome. My biggest concern was her weight loss, which did not seem to bother her. She worked for a nutritional supplement company that espoused "weight management and healthy living," something the employees had to embody. As a result, she considered her weight natural.

I evaluated her for food allergies and parasites of the gastrointestinal tract. The exam yielded the following diagnosis. It turned out she not only had a chronic fatigue syndrome caused by a derangement of her adrenal system, but I also found worms and other parasites in her GI tract. As we discussed her condition, she mentioned she had traveled to India and Asia and the surrounding countries many times, and was frequently exposed to a non-Western diet. We agreed that this was probably the cause of the worms and parasites.

I prescribed her an antiparasitic agent and recommended correcting the adrenal fatigue aggravated by chronic diarrhea with some natural supplements and an adrenal gland rebuilder. A few weeks later, I got a call at the office. She was calling me from somewhere in Asia to tell me that after ten years of pain and discomfort the diarrhea had finally stopped, and she felt more energetic and better than ever.

Please refer to the website www.gotpaindocs.com, www.thegreatPainJack.com, or www. thegreatPainJack.org, for further information.

Case Study: *I serve as a civilian field pain management referral specialist for the USS "Aircraft Carrier to remain nameless," an aircraft carrier with a population of about five thousand. Since there is no medical specialist for pain management onboard, and only a nurse anesthetist and flight surgeon to address medical concerns, I occasionally handle medical issues remotely by e-mail while this ship is abroad and on duty.*

One particular e-mail caught my interest. It involved Dale, a young serviceman who had injured his groin. The nurse anesthetist believed that he had incurred neuralgia of the ilio-inguinal nerve. He asked me about the likelihood of this condition. I told him that the possibilities of neuralgia of this sort are not uncommon, especially after hernia repair. Occasionally, during the sewing of the mesh material during the repair of a hernia, a branch of one of the nerves gets trapped in the scar tissue. The entrapped nerve becomes irritated as the scar contracts and pulls the nerve inwards.

I quickly e-mailed instructions for the proper dosing of injections for Dale, and, though the ship was somewhere in the Middle East, my e-mail was received within seconds. The injection technique and dosing information that travelled thousands of miles was quickly relayed to the anesthetist, who promptly injected the medication into the injured serviceman. Within minutes of my receipt of the original e-mail request, Dale was pain-free.

Acute abdominal pain must be dealt with much quicker than chronic pain. If surgery is required, the surgeon may recommend an exploratory incision into the abdomen to make a diagnosis. Abdominal problems can be life-threatening and should be diagnosed and treated very carefully. Abdominal pain should clearly be differentiated from urologic and gynecologic symptoms.

> **Case Study:** *I was covering at a local hospital, which was transitioning its anesthesia care team. Rich in resources, the hospital served an important role in the care of the elderly and the poor in its community. One of the hospital's frequent visitors was Kellie, a young, obese, female patient, well-known by the operating room and GI staff. She suffered from an unusual disorder, which would result in a trip to the operating room on a weekly, sometimes biweekly basis.*

Her problem was that she would eat things. Inedible things. Plastic knives and forks, rolled tape, socks, coins, underwear, cassettes, iPods, plastic bottles, and other items. I never quite understood how this clearly disturbed woman managed to swallow some of these things whole, but in my short time at the institution I witnessed at least seven different retrieval procedures performed on her.

The skilled gastroenterologist would enter the mouth of her gastrointestinal tract using an endoscope and retrieve the object, which was typically lodged in the stomach or below in the intestines. Fortunately, the items were retrieved via endoscopy before doing extensive damage to the gastrointestinal tract. I recommended referral to a psychiatrist to treat the underlying mental issues that, if untreated, would keep bringing Kellie back to the emergency room for the same procedure.

Occasionally, plastic surgery like abdominoplasty or a tummy tuck can result in pain related to an initial strain of the abdominal muscles. This strain can become chronic. This condition can be further complicated by a bacterial infection known as MRSA (*methicillin-resistant staphylococcus sureus*). It is very hard to treat, the healing process is complex, and it delays the healing of the abdominal wall. Furthermore, when the abdominal musculature is stretched too tight or the tissue has become too thin, it can remain in a state of constant spasm.

I have a few patients who have suffered from this. Occasionally muscle relaxants and analgesics will relieve the milder cases of pain. For the more severe ones, an abdominal ultrasound may be successful. Additionally, the abdominal musculature can be blocked with needle injections of long-acting local anesthetic and steroid. If these blocks fail to relieve the condition, advanced pain therapies can be implemented such as neuromodulation and/or intrathecal pump implant for intractable cases.

> **Case Study:** *I was once asked by a surgeon colleague to treat Mr. N——, a very famous singer in Los Angeles, who was suffering from a complication after a tummy tuck. Apparently the abdominal binder worn after the procedure was so tight it constricted the blood flow to the healing tissue. This resulted in a small area of dead tissue. Because the consequences were more cosmetic rather than functional, an abdominal ultrasound and analgesics were*

enough to bring about healing of the condition. As a result, the singer did not miss any tour dates or recording sessions.

My colleague was relieved to hear that his patient did not develop a chronic pain condition and was extremely happy that he did not get sued.

Case Study: *After a tummy tuck, Mrs. G—— was referred to me for treatment of pain and spasm in her abdominal wall. I ordered a CAT scan, an MRI, and an ultrasound, but all three failed to reveal anything of note except some slight bending in the abdominal wall, near the scar from the surgical procedure.*

Despite severe abdominal pain and daily spasms, Mrs. G—— maintained a very positive outlook. Nevertheless, her pain was often so extreme she would double over and not be able to function for hours.

After careful diagnosis I determined that she suffered from a poorly understood but not uncommon condition known as cutaneous neuroma formation. Sometimes, after plastic surgery like a tummy tuck, this painful syndrome can develop. Basically, when the abdominal muscles are stretched too tight they can remain in a state of constant spasm. This can lead to the development of an autoimmune dysfunction, like cutaneous neuroma formation. It's also very difficult to treat. It involves painful nerve tangles that attempt to reconnect with each other. The condition is related to an initial strain of the abdominal muscles, and can become chronic. Worse, it can lead to the formation of antibodies to the muscles involved in the entanglement. Essentially, the antibodies begin to perceive the body's own tissue as foreign, and they recruit other cells in an attempt to destroy it.

Needless to say, Mrs. G—— took great comfort in knowing the reason behind her pain. While abdominal spasms are difficult to treat because we use our abdominal muscles constantly, I prescribed her celiac plexus block injections that healed her condition.

Please refer to the website www.gotpaindocs.com, www.thegreatPainJack.com, or www. thegreatPainJack.org for further information.

Case Study: *A successful software engineer, Mrs. C—— was a very young woman with a history of pancreatitis and abnormalities of the liver and gallbladder. She came to see me not because of these problems, however, but because she developed a chronic pain syndrome that interfered with her daily activities, including her job.*

She'd seen multiple gastroenterologists, who had performed multiple procedures and multiple tests on her gallbladder, liver, and pancreas. A stent was placed in the ducts of her liver, but the procedure also damaged an important structure in the liver. She was transferred to another institution for a second stent procedure. She started to lose weight, stopped being able to eat without vomiting, and started taking over 50 mg of hydromorphone a day.

When she came to see me, we tried a celiac plexus injection to block the pain arising from her stomach. After the injection, she felt immediate relief, but it lasted only four hours. I decided to go a step further and prescribed a delicate balance of narcotics, muscle relaxants, and other tranquilizers, including antidepressants.

However, the pain continued unabated, as did her weight loss. I tried an injection of spinal narcotic and admitted her to the hospital for overnight observation. The next twenty-four hours were unbelievable. Her pain diminished, and her appetite returned completely. She ate without any difficulties.

Since the procedure was successful, I decided that a more permanent solution would involve a permanent intrathecal pump. The pump is a device about the size of a hockey puck, placed in or around the abdomen, and attached to a catheter that delivers a premeasured amount of narcotic directly into the patient's spinal fluid.

Mrs. C—— had an excellent experience with implantation therapy. She has to get her pump filled once every six months, which allowed her to reduce her medication and her visits to the doctor. Most importantly, she experiences only minimal pain now and rarely at that.

Case Study: Mr. S—— would experience severe muscle spasms after intense abdominal workouts. He continued his exercise routine but, despite multiple interventions, never experienced any relief. These interventions included abdominal injections, which helped control symptoms of his condition; however, his pain typically returned four to six weeks later.

He was very young, in great shape, and was baffling to his doctor who, after ordering a barrage of tests, could not confirm a diagnosis. Finally, a celiac plexus block injection along with intramuscular injections to his abdominal muscles brought him relief.

I still could not confirm why Mr. S—— had abnormal spasms. I sent him to undergo a specialty workout at a university center, which yielded interesting results. It turns out that he had antibodies that developed to the striated muscle cells within the abdominal wall. His may have been a genetic condition, but an environmental trigger could have been responsible as well for the body's rejection of its own muscle cells. Please refer to the website www. gotpaindocs.com, www.thegreatPainJack.com, or www.thegreatPainJack.org, for further information.

Abdominal Pain Questionnaire—Answer these questions to map pain symptoms

*(Copy and fill out these worksheets and bring to your doctor. He/she may have his/her own, but answers to these questions provide a good overview of your pain condition and will help you remember and collect a **pain profile** in order to use your time with your doctor more effectively.)*

Where is your pain located? _____

In what part of the abdomen does the pain seem to be most prominent? _____

Is it also in your pelvis? _____

When does your pain start and end? _____

Is it related to mealtime? _____

Does it occur one hour after eating? _____

When did you first begin to have abdominal pain, to the best of your recollection?

Where does your abdominal pain travel to? _____

Is it continuous throughout the day? _____

Has your abdominal pain ever improved? _____

Is it relieved with bowel movements? _____

Has it become chronic? _____

Is it associated with nausea and vomiting? _____

Could there be two or more different types of pain syndromes that seem to occur simultaneously? _____

Does your abdominal pain wax and wane, or does it stay at the same intensity throughout the course of the day? _____

Does the pain occur all over your body as well as in the abdomen? _____

Which abdominal pain bothers you the most? _____

Does eating or fasting help the abdominal pain get better? _____

Do you have a systemic disease diagnosed previously that may be contributing to your abdominal pain? _____

Perhaps celiac sprue (gluten intolerance) or perhaps lactose intolerance? _____

Do you have a history of cancer of any abdominal or pelvic organs? _____

Have you had hepatitis before? _____

Do you have a history of heavy drinking? _____

Any history of bleeding from the gastrointestinal tract, including vomiting or spitting up dark blood? _____

Do you believe your abdominal pain is caused by accident or injury? _____ _____

Could this abdominal pain have begun as a work-related injury? _____

Does your abdominal pain feel like a muscle ache? _____

Could an old injury that did not heal be exacerbated by current daily activities? _____ _____

Use the following scale to describe the severity of your pain for each type of pain you have, with 1 being the least amount of pain and 10 being the highest level of pain you could ever imagine: 1 … 2 … 3 … 4 … 5 … 6 … 7 … 8 … 9 … 10.

What descriptors can you use for your pain: Burning? Aching? Shooting? Sharp? Throbbing? Cramping? Constant? Numbing? Lancinating? Stabbing? Transient? Excruciating? Tingling? On fire?

Does your pain get worse or better with sitting, bending, lifting, walking, grasping, sweeping, standing, crawling, squatting, reaching overhead, eating, coughing, sneezing, physical activity, stress, driving, sexual intercourse, heat, ice, physical therapy, medications?

Have any of the following treatments provided relief of your pain condition: Surgery? Medications? Injection therapy? Chiropractic? Tens unit (electric stimulation)? Physical therapy? Traction? Heat therapy? Bed rest? Acupuncture? Psychotherapy? _____

Specific questions regarding abdominal pain to best allow you and your doctor to make a diagnosis

Does the pain seem to arise in the midabdomen or lower part of the abdomen? _____ Could it be referred to the abdomen?

Is the abdominal pain fleeting, transient, or intermittent? Does it come in waves or cycles? Is the pain constant and/or throbbing? _____ Is the pain sharp?

Is the abdominal pain associated with a vascular phenomenon? menstrual periods? premenstrual syndrome? _____ sexual function?

Is the abdominal pain associated with: Numbness or tingling? _____ Weakness of any of the muscles of the abdomen? _____ Paralysis? _____ Increased or decreased sweating? Skin discoloration? Skin rash anywhere on the body? Tingling pins and needles on the face or body? _____ Cold? _____ Muscle spasm tightness? _____ Trouble sleeping? "Touch me not" pain? _____

Is there a history of sexually transmitted disease or urologic dysfunction? _____

Is there a history of food allergies? _____ Is there a history of Crohn's disease or ulcerative colitis? _____

Is there a history of pancreatic disease or cancer? _____ Is there a history of diabetes? _____

What improves your abdominal pain? _____ What medications have you tried that failed? Have you had injections for your abdominal pain? _____ Celiac plexus nerve block? Other type of spinal or other type of injection? _____

What specifically helps your abdominal pain: Sleep? _____ Rest? Ice? _____ Heat? Pressure? Exercise? _____ Any type of therapy? _____ Any kind of surgery? _____ Have you used light or laser therapy to try to treat your abdominal pain? _____

What specific medications have you tried that failed? _____

What specific herbal or natural remedies have you tried? _____

Do you take supplements for your condition? _____

Is your abdominal pain accompanied with transient paralysis? _____ Do the muscles of your body go into spasm or become distorted at any time? _____ Do the abdominal muscles appear to be weaker at any time? _____

Body Map for Abdominal Pain Questionnaire

Figure 6A
Abdominal Pain

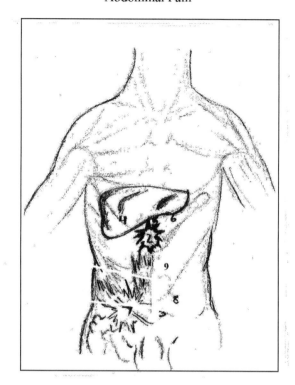

1. Cutaneous Nerve Entrapment Syndrome
2. Acute Intermittent Porphyria
3. Radiation Enteritis
4. Liver Pain
5. Abdominal Angina
6. Pancreatitis
7. Ilioinguinal Neuralgia
8. Genitofemoral Neuralgia
9. Cancer

Figue 7B
Abdominal Pain

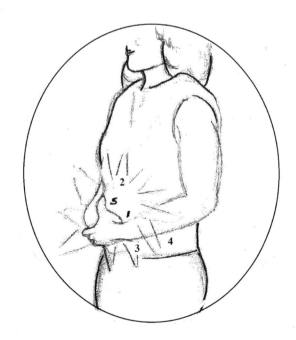

1. Liver Pain
2. Radiation Enteritis
3. Acute Intermittent Porphyria
4. Cancer
5. Abdominal Angina

Chapter 8:

So, You've Got Obstetric Pain?

Despite being referred to as a "miracle," giving birth is often associated with extreme pain—pain of going into labor, pain of giving birth, and/or pain during a C-section, not to mention postoperative pain due to swelling and other possible obstetric and gynecological problems. In fact, a comparison of pain scores in a recent review revealed that the degree of labor pain ranged between that of cancer pain and the amputation of a digit.

On top of the naturally attendant physical suffering, fear and anxiety may contribute to labor pain in some women. As a result, preparation for childbirth now focuses on both the physical and psychological factors involved. For instance, studies have shown that proper childbirth prep can decrease the amount of anesthetic and analgesic drugs used during labor and delivery. Additionally, in a well-prepared mother, childbirth is more likely to be an enjoyable experience that may strengthen the maternal bond with the child. Interestingly, studies have also shown that a father's preparation and increased participation in the birth process may play an important role in reducing overall analgesia in the mother as well.

A number of different "psychological" anesthesias have been used with varying degrees of success. These include hypnosis, "natural childbirth," and "psychoprophylaxis." Other methods include acupuncture and the LeBoyer technique, as well as transcutaneous electrical nerve stimulation. These techniques have been used independently and in combination with anesthesia, depending on the requirements of the mother in question.

Nonchemical Anesthetic Methods

Hypnosis

Hypnosis has been used for pain relief in childbirth for many years. The hypnotic trance achieves the analgesic, painkiller effect with no depressant effect on the baby or the mother. Also, several studies have found that hypnosis can shorten labor. Hypnosis is not always effective and not without risk to some women, especially those with a history of psychosis. In my experience, most women request epidural anesthesia for labor discomfort for vaginal deliveries and epidural or intraspinal anesthesia for cesarean section.

Natural Childbirth

The term "natural childbirth" was widely used in the 1940s. It is now recognized as having significant limitations. The basis of this approach was the fact that anxiety, fear, and pain were interlinked, the fear and anxiety stemming from the complexity of the procedure. Thus, it was believed that a simplified approach to labor could render it painless. Grantly Dick-Read, the originator of the theory, believed that during uncomplicated labor uterine contractions should be painless because "there is no physiological function of the body which gives rise to pain in the normal course of health."

Psychoprophylaxis

The psychoprophylactic method, introduced by a doctor named Lamaze, is currently one of the most popular approaches; it consists of several relaxation techniques. The basis of the psychoprophylaxis is the belief that the pain of labor and delivery can be suppressed by reorganization of brain activity. The mother is taught to respond to contractions by taking a deep "cleansing breath" and gently exhaling, breathing in a specific pattern until the contractions end. She also focuses her eyes on a specific object or location away from herself. This allows her to concentrate on the release of muscle tension and to maintain the proper breathing rhythm.

The level of concentration these exercises require of the mother distracts her from or inhibits the pain she may feel. This method usually begins six weeks before delivery. A coach instructs the mothers (and their partners) in the anatomy and physiology of their pregnancy, labor, and delivery, providing them with knowledge and understanding of the process they are undergoing.

Nevertheless, as with hypnosis, a majority of women receiving Lamaze training will often request additional anesthesia during labor, since excessive pain or anxiety during labor may result in harm to the fetus. Also, researchers Myers and Morishima have demonstrated that a mother's psychological stress during labor may reduce oxygen flow to the fetus. On the other hand, since certain types and amounts of analgesic and anesthetic drugs injected into the mother may also sedate the fetus, an argument can be made against chemical anesthesia for childbirth. The reasonable compromise involves the use of regional anesthesia, which minimizes stress but allows the participation of the mother and father in the birthing process.

In the end, the Lamaze method is a benefit to almost all women and, regardless if anesthesia is used, can make the experience of childbirth more pleasant.

Acupuncture

Acupuncture has been practiced in China for more than a thousand years due to its therapeutic and painkilling properties. Anecdotal reports have created interest in the value of acupuncture as an alternative to conventional anesthesia. The interest can be partially explained by the fact that the method seems completely safe for the mother and the newborn. In China, acupuncture anesthesia during surgery is reported to be successful in about 70 percent of patients. However, this number depends on careful patient selection, high patient motivation, and inherent cultural conditioning. In an American study, when several doctors used acupuncture as a painkiller during labor, nineteen out of the twenty-one patients complained of inadequate analgesia.

LeBoyer Technique

The French obstetrician Frederick O. LeBoyer has received significant attention for promoting the concept of "childbirth without violence." He believed that the noise, bright lights, and other stimulation associated with traditional delivery caused psychological trauma to the newborn. His solution was to perform deliveries in near silence and semidarkness, which minimized the newborn's crying. LeBoyer would then place the newborn on the mother's abdomen with the umbilical cord still attached and pulsating. According to his theory, this process would diminish the potential psychological "violence" done to an infant during its birth.

Transcutaneous Electrical Nerve Stimulation (TENS)

The use of electricity for analgesia dates to the ancient Greeks and Romans, who would use the torpedo fish, which can emit 200 volts, to kill pain. Although the use of electricity in modern medicine has been erratic and not always safe, developments in the field of electronics, such as TENS, have posed an interesting alternative to conventional means of analgesia. TENS works by shutting down an area in the central nervous system known as *substantia gelatinosa* (located in the spinal cord), through which pain sensations normally travel to the brain. When this area, or gate, is closed, these sensations theoretically do not reach the brain. Unfortunately, there are few well-controlled studies performed, with little reliable information available.

In general, TENS pain relief is most successful during the first stage of labor and is diminished by the second stage. Also, when TENS is implemented, the use of narcotics during labor decreases. The major drawback to TENS is that the unit can create electrical interference with the fetal heart rate monitoring system, although it has no effect on the fetal heart rate itself, or the EKG.

Not too long ago, at the turn of the twentieth century, childbearing was associated with at least a 10 percent mortality rate. This means that one in ten women would die during the birthing process due to various complications.

This mortality rate is unacceptable today in the Western world. With the use of modern monitoring tools, including antepartum testing, routine ultrasound checks, amniocentesis, evaluation for different proteins, and other testing, abnormalities of a pregnancy can be detected earlier. The implementation of modern anesthetic techniques and proper birth planning have significantly reduced maternal and infant mortality, to currently less than 1 percent in the United States.

Case Study: It was a hot summer night, and I was doing an obstetric call at a community hospital. I had finished my usual scheduled C-sections and deliveries around 11:30 p.m. I told myself I was going to luck out with an easy call, with no emergency deliveries or C-sections in the middle of the night.

A phone call broke me out of my reverie. It was around 2:30 a.m. I picked it up and was informed by a hospital staff member that I was urgently needed to place a breathing tube in a very small premature baby that had been delivered minutes earlier.

When I arrived at the scene, I could not believe my eyes. The infant weighed less than three pounds and was smaller than my palm. It was about twenty-five weeks, about three months premature. The respiratory team was trying to place a breathing tube in the tiny mouth to begin resuscitation but couldn't do it. Without it, this twenty-five-week-old infant would die, its lungs too immature to oxygenate the small body on their own.

I managed to open the baby's mouth, which was about as big as my thumbnail. I used a device known as a laryngoscope to open its airway and, almost blindly, inserted a breathing tube to where I thought the opening of the trachea was. After that, the infant was successfully resuscitated.

Chemical Anesthetic Methods and C-Sections

To eliminate pain during the laboring process, different anesthetic techniques and types of management have been employed. In the 1800s, aside from a spinal injection of anesthetic, mask inhalation of ether was used to reduce pain in delivery. In some cultures, such as in Haiti, a brew made from tea leaves is utilized as anesthesia. In certain Asian countries other herbs and naturally occurring substances are used for the same effect. Also, there are other cultural considerations in the approach to pain of the laboring process. For instance, pain tolerance has been linked not only to genetic backgrounds but also to a mother's upbringing. Certainly, an argument can be made for adequacy of a mother's birthing hips and her ability to deliver larger infants with relative ease.

In the West, in the past two decades it has been commonplace to administer epidural anesthesia to a patient on demand. The *epidural catheter* is a thin plastic tube used to deliver a pain-relieving medication, which is placed inside the patient. This blocks the sensory nerves from sending a pain signal to the brain. However, if a potentially catastrophic event was to occur during the birthing process, like an imminent uterine rupture, the blocked pain signal would be overwritten, and pain would not be suppressed, alerting the patient and the obstetrician.

In an era of medical legal practice, an obstetrician will often opt for a very quick C-Section to avoid complications instead of delivering the baby vaginally. For a new mother, a C-section assures that the woman will be destined to undergo cesarean sections for all future deliveries. The decision was primarily set forth as a result of guidelines established by the American College of Obstetricians and Gynecologists (ACOG). This group found that a significant number of adverse outcomes were occurring in alarming frequency when women were allowed to proceed with vaginal birth after prior C-section. This has led to an increase in C-sections across the nation in the last decade.

In America today very few obstetricians will take the risk of accommodating vaginal birth after C-section (VBAC) patients. Should a mother want vaginal delivery after a C-section, she would need to make arrangements with her local hospital in advance to make sure an emergency team is continuously available on standby once labor begins. This again is primarily due to the safety recommendations of ACOG.

Fetal distress usually manifests itself as an abnormal neonatal heart rate. As anesthesiologists, we are trained to listen to tones that bear a certain frequency when measuring various vital signs. An astute anesthesiologist or obstetrician will know just by the change in tone of the pulse oximeter how well a mother or a baby is doing.

Measurement of oxygen saturation percent is a management tool that has brought about great change in safety in the delivery of all anesthetics in the last twenty years. The pulse oximeter, which measures it, is such a valuable tool that it is considered a standard monitor.

> **Case Study:** *I was called in the middle of the night to provide an anesthetic to a pregnant woman experiencing fetal distress. Debra had had three prior C-sections, which, her obstetrician believed, had thinned out the wall of her uterus. Indeed, the risk for uterine rupture is higher among women with prior C-sections than among those without. Furthermore, without careful monitoring of delivery, the woman's chance of having an adverse outcome is significantly increased.*
>
> *At first things appeared very normal. At 2:00 a.m., however, your sense of awareness heightens, and mine was telling me that something was very off. I quickly placed a spinal anesthetic through a needle to numb Debra below the waistline. When I retracted the needle, the little hole I had made in the skin began bleeding profusely, even though the needle I used, a 25-gauge, was tiny.*
>
> *Because of the fetal distress, the C-section proceeded without further delay, and a magnificent eight-and-a-half-pound girl emerged. Intravenous fluids were administered to the mother to counter the rather excessive loss of blood that occurred during the procedure.*

Since the new mom was awake during the C-section and had been doing extremely well, with no indications of blood instability, there was no reason to call the blood bank. I rolled to the postanesthesia recovery area at 3:00 a.m., deliriously happy with the baby girl's delivery.

An hour later, the recovery room nurses came in and told me that the mother was still bleeding from her vagina, and her blood pressure was dropping. Within minutes of the call, I arrived in the recovery room and found that her pressure had dropped to an extremely low 70/40. Her heart rate wasn't any better, rapidly pulsating at 150.

These were grave vital signs for someone that had been given aggressive fluids to counteract her intraoperative loss of blood. The blood dripped onto the gurney, trickling down to the floor. Debra appeared completely pale and did not say much. Suddenly, her body started to convulse. She appeared to be having grand mal seizures. It was time to act quickly and dramatically.

The lab was summoned immediately. A complete blood count and various other tests were ordered. Four units of blood were administered through an intravenous line I inserted into a large vein in the neck. I ordered three more liters, and by 5:00 a.m. the situation seemed to be improving.

The seizures complicated her diagnosis. I suspected preeclampsia, a condition affecting women that results in increased blood pressure, abnormal neurological signs, and generalized swelling and edema, which can lead to seizures. Because the patient was monitored with the oxygen saturation device, I was able to rule out brain seizures caused by lack of oxygen.

As the fluids entered her veins, the seizures became quiescent. Her blood pressure increased to over 100 on the systolic scale for the first time in two hours. The heart rate returned close to normal, and the hemorrhaging ceased. Her condition stabilized.

I dragged myself back to the on-call hospital room only to hear my 5:30 a.m. alarm clock ring for the beginning of a new day.

Chapter 9:

So, You've Got Pelvic Pain?

Case Study: *Mrs. G—— noted that she had vaginal pain that occurred most of the time. She had been told by her gynecologist that there was nothing wrong with her. She continued to struggle with determining if the condition was in her head. A series of complex studies indicated that indeed her condition was "not in her head." We embarked on a course of bioidentical hormone replacement and evaluation for lumbar degenerative disc disease. After replacing hormones and performing epidural injections for degenerative disc disease, her vaginal pain and overall health and feelings of well-being improved dramatically*

Generally disorders of pelvic and gynecologic pain can be grouped into a number of categories. The enervation of the pelvis is through the abdominal and visceral nerves, which provide input into the spinal cord and then relay the information up to the brain, where the brain can interpret the signal and provide a response. Some of these conditions can masquerade as symptoms of abdominal pain. Pathologies, some of which have been previously described, are related to gynecologic and reproductive system abnormalities. Such conditions, including tumors of the ovaries and/or uterus, as well as benign fibroid and benign cystic formation in the ovaries, are generally the more common pain conditions. Rarely torsion of the ovary, which is a flipping of the ovary in the abdominal mesentery, can also provide pelvic pain in the female. Please refer to the website www.gotpaindocs.com for further information.

Other conditions that are known to occur with relative frequency in the female include *osteitis pubis*, which is a painful inflammation of the bone in the pubis region, *piriformis syndrome*, and *bursitis* of the ischio-gluteal and coccydynia, which is pain in the tailbone. Other conditions that are known to be painful are *orchealgia* and *prostadynia*, which is a constellation of disorders that can cause pain in the anatomic region of the prostate. This condition includes the chronic inflammation of the prostate without infection, bladder outflow abnormalities, reflex-synthetic dystrophy, pelvic muscle disorders, and psychogenic causes. There is in all of these entities a chronic, ill-defined, and perineal pain, which is the hallmark of prostadynia. Typically the pain is characterized by a dull aching or burning in the perinea and underlining structures. The worsening of the pain may occur with urination and sexual activity. The pain of prostadynia may be referred to pain in the testicles, scrotum, or the inner thigh region. There may be urinary outflow symptoms and sexual dysfunction may coexist with the pain.

The treatment should be directed at identifying the acute bacterial infection of the prostate or urinary tract. If there is acute orchitis, or inflammation of the testicles, secondary to infections, these patients will usually have an exquisitely tender prostate. Sometimes they will experience a symptom known as allodynia of the perineal area. This condition is extremely intolerant to any touch whatsoever. Prostate cancer should always be considered in patients complaining of prostate pain, although the first symptoms of prostate cancer are typically nonpainful.

One of the most common causes of the painful prostate is malignancy of the pelvic contents other than the prostate, involving the nerve area known as the lumbar plexus. Postradiation aropathy after radiation therapy of treatment of the cancer also can mimic as prostadynia. Ultrasound examination of the prostate and digital examination is the cornerstone plan of the treatment of these conditions. MRI or CT scanning is also recommended. Urine analysis should also be conducted to look for bacteria.

Initial treatment of prostadynia should include anti-inflammatory nonsteroidal medication, and antibiotic therapy may be effective. Occasionally some patients have been found to respond to hariponol, a drug used to treat gout.

Generally disorders of the pelvis should be separated into pain coming from the spine region and areas surrounding the tailbone, and pain coming from the lower abdominal region and pelvis. Occasionally differentiating between the two is difficult. A diagnostic test and a physical exam are helpful in making this examination. The area that is most exquisitely tender is usually the first to test. Most of these conditions do not predispose to chronic pain; however, in chronic pain conditions that are deemed to be greater than three months, a workup should be formulated.

The diagnostic blocks may be performed after CT and MRIs have not provided an accurate diagnosis. For example, bursitis that is located on the underside of the buttocks may be best approached with an injection of local anesthetic as well as long-lasting steroids.

Because the sciatic nerve may travel anatomically above or below the piriformis muscle, piriformis syndrome can predispose to a painful gait as well as to a buttock that hurts. Differential injections combined with a rectal examination will provide an accurate diagnosis of piriformis syndrome. Generally, severe pain on the side that is affected is a good indicator of the syndrome. The anatomical variation of the syndrome can be seen with the variability of the nerve passage over and under the muscle.

Pelvic pain can also have gynecologic origin, best diagnosed by a gynecologist. If appropriate, ultrasound studies along with MRIs should be performed to rule out structure abnormalities such as cysts on the ovaries or fibroids. Fibroids are typically benign enlargements of the uterus or growths stemming from hormones. Pelvic inflammatory disease can be of a chronic nature and be related to a scarring of the fallopian tubes as well as generalized pain of the abdominal and pelvic regions.

Please refer to the website www.gotpaindocs.com for further information.

Coccydynia is simply tailbone pain, which can be initiated by previous trauma, such as coccyx or tailbone fracture. A painful syndrome may develop. It can be treated with ganglion impars injection into the inside portion of the nerve, coalescing on the innermost portion of the tailbone.

I've had at least one patient who has undergone specific treatment for tailbone pain. One such patient, a woman, had a tremendous amount of treatments and surgeries including a disk replacement surgery, all of which did not relieve her condition. A partial reconstruction of the tailbone has been suggested, but she has been reluctant to this day to pursue this course, and we continue to treat her with injections.

Chronic pelvic pain can be very difficult to fully treat. Conditions of chronic nature may or may not respond to injection therapy. But the implication on gait exercise and sexual function is paramount. These can cause peripheral pain in individuals suffering from this, interrupting their daily lives. If the diagnosis can be reached early, then these conditions may be prevented from becoming chronic, thereby stopping them from spreading pain into other body parts. When other nerve systems are entwined in the diagnosis, things become very convoluted, and it becomes difficult to sort out which symptoms belong to which constellation of disease process.

Screening for malignancies should always occur. This should always be at the back of a physician's mind. However, since pain is not the first symptom of cancer, this is very hard to do. Endomitrial cancer is a very curable disease, but unfortunately it is difficult to diagnose. Postmenopausal bleeding is a symptom, and in a postmenopausal woman bleeding should be considered related to cancer until the possibility is ruled out. Unfortunately, women have died with improper diagnoses of early endomitrial cancer. If this cancer is able to pierce the wall of the uterus after its symptoms have been noted, then cure can be unlikely. A cure, as a last resort, would involve the removal of the uterus and its surrounding structures. However, if the diseased cells pass the inside lining of the uterus, then the surgical cure is much less likely.

Treatments range from antibiotics, anti-inflammatory medication, narcotic analgesics, and, of course, surgery.

Case Sudy A divorced twenty-eight-year-old woman comes to complain about interstitial cystitis. She says she has given up her career in occupational and physical medicine to be able to raise her two small children and manage her pain. Her pain syndrome arises from an inflammatory bladder condition. The hallmarks include urinary urgency, frequency, and severe pain. It is not uncommon that these patients have to urinate up to fifty times during a twenty-four-hour period. This woman's case can also be combined with the case of another person who suffered from the same thing. Both patients went through the pelvic floor therapy program. This is an evaluation of the pelvic pain generator and a physical therapy course whereby the pelvic floor muscles are taught to relax and thwart the symptoms of the condition.

Both individuals had seen their gynecologist prior to coming to me, and I might add that gynecologists are ill-prepared to deal with interstitial cystitis and similar pelvic pain syndromes, which should be referred out to pain management specialists. The gynecologic training is not suitable to treating this type of condition, particularly the comorbid conditions that are known to occur, such as irritable bowel syndrome, endometriosis, generalized pain due to floor dysfunction, and fibromyalgia. All of these conditions indicate that there may be a neuropathic or pain component coming from the nerves themselves.

Of the people I treated, one was offered a spinal cord simulator finally, and she obtained excellent relief from her condition. The other young woman, who's still undergoing treatment, chose medications as a treatment plan.

Interstitial Cystitis

Interstitial cystitis was discovered in 1915 by Guy Hunner, who evaluated these conditions and saw ulcers on the bladder wall. Urologists at the time and through today considered this disorder to be psychosomatic because there has been no diagnostic test to determine interstitial cystitis. Urologic textbooks in the 1970s and '80s have described it as an emotional disorder.

Diagnosis and Treatment

Hopeful diagnostic studies in treating interstitial cystitis discover a protein in the urine of patients with this condition. This specific protein is called an antiproliforative factor. Its presence indicates that there happens to be some damage to the lining of the bladder, which causes this protein to be secreted into the urine.

Classic interstitial cystitis, described as Hunner's lesions, on the bladder wall are ulcers that occur and can be diagnosed through laparoscopy. It is diagnosed based on a constellation of symptoms and excluding other conditions that produce similar symptoms, such as urinary tract infection and cancer of the bladder.

In a recent survey of one hundred thousand US households using symptom-based definitions, it was revealed that 3 to 8 percent of women could be afflicted with this condition. The number of men is less certain.

Because the pain and dysfunction and loss of work and sexual function affect so many people's lives, this syndrome can be considered as severe as end-stage kidney disease.

Women who suffer from interstitial cystitis experience sleep loss, sexual dysfunction, and depression.

Other sources of pain from this condition include the pelvic floor muscle dysfunction, irritable bowel syndrome (IBS) allergies, vulvadynia (painful vulva), endometriosis, pudendal neuralgia, fibromyalgia, and depression. There has been evidence of neurogenic inflammation between the bowel and bladder, also between visceral organs and skin.

Since fibromyalgia is a commonly associated syndrome, sensitization plays an important role in interstitial cystitis. This has historically led people to believe that it was a psychosomatic disorder. Because of the interrelationship between the body, the bladder, visceral organs, and the skin, a recruitment of other neurons and nerve tracks has also been suggested. Thus, cornerstones of treatment focus on neuroleptic and topical medications and the elimination of dietary foods that promote this dysfunction. Food allergies are common among people who suffer from pelvic pain.

Oral medication therapy focuses around medications such as elmiron, which is a medication specifically approved for interstitial cystitis, theorized to restore a part of the bladder, thus preventing the ulcers that are known to occur in the bladder. Other medications known to help treat this are amitryptaline, which is a tricyclic antidepressant. This tricyclic antidepressant medication is helpful because of its sedative effects, promoting sleep and alleviating pain accompanying urination. Antispasmodic medications thought to improve an overactive bladder are generally not helpful. Symptoms can be abated if these medications are also used.

Hydrodistension, or the instilling of fluid in the bladder, may reduce symptoms. Laser treatments and fulguration with an electrode, burning the lesions off the bladder, all surgical procedures, have also helped.

Other types of therapies are avoidance of certain triggers, which can worsen symptoms, such as caffeine, tea, sodas, artificial sweeteners, citrus fruit, tomatoes, and tomato products. This can improve symptoms. Commonly urologists will instill anesthetic cocktails into the bladder. The common agent for this is dimethylsulfoxide, otherwise known as DMSO. Please see www.got.paindocs.com, www.thegreatPainJack.com, or www.thegreatPainJack. org for more information.

Most universal treatments for interstitial cystitis are based on a small series of tests and anecdotal reports. The Interstitial Cystitis Association, which is dedicated to promoting information about and treatment of this disorder, was formed. Most physicians that treat IC realize that a multimodal methodology is appropriate. However, an individualized approach is often necessary.

Some of the problems of treatment of IC, include the doctor not realizing that endometriosis or vulvadynia, powerful pain generators, are occurring and need to be treated simultaneously and separately. A gynecologist or an obstetrician may not realize that the bladder is the main pain generator. Both of these specialists forget that the bowel may also play a part in causing pain. This should not be overlooked in the constellation of symptoms.

Tenderness generating from the pelvic floor muscle can be responsible for as much as 80 percent of the pain in patients suffering from IC. Simple things such as exercise and sexual activity can create severe pelvic pain. Treating pelvic floor pain may be a very effective method of dealing with IC, including with intravaginal injections of valium, which can also improve sexual function by relaxing the pelvic muscle. Doctors that prescribe topical analgesics have been findings that application to the supra of the pubic region can relieve some of the symptoms. Trigger-point injections used and combined with anesthetics into the pelvic floor can alleviate some of the spasmodic symptoms of IC. A fluoroscope-guided plexus block can be used as well.

Case Study *A young man was referred to me once. His visit was striking in that he, at thirty-four, came to the office with a cane. It was unclear as to how this young man, formerly a soccer player, had come to sustain such an injury. He explained to me that he was once a passenger in a car that sustained a rear-end impact collision.*

Prior to the car accident he had a light swelling in his groin, and he was due to see the doctor at some point in the future. He apparently scheduled an appointment three months from the car accident. He stated that after the accident he developed extreme groin swelling and tenderness. He said that as time progressed and hospital care was denied for treatment of his condition (presumably hernia), his pain, dysfunction, and feelings of futility increased.

This unfortunate man was not able to see any physician in the area because he did not have health insurance. Since an attorney contacted my office regarding his care, I agreed to see the patient, even though hernial repair was not my immediate specialty. The patient was worked up with an MRI, an ultrasound of his scrotum and groin, as well as a CAT scan of the abdomen and pelvis. He did sustain some injuries, but chest and rib x-rays were reported as negative.

After diagnosis was made and examination was performed, I told the patient that I would not be immediately able to find a surgeon who would operate on his hernia. I contacted numerous colleagues of mine who were general surgeons, indicating that I had a likely candidate for hernia repair. One by one, they started saying no.

As the list dwindled to a few remaining surgeons that might accept this patient and perform this surgery, I was losing hope in the medical system. My despair and futility grew as I realized that I could not find a surgeon who would treat this individual within a 250-mile radius of his home city.

Finally, I contacted one of my colleagues in a local county of California who agreed to see the patient on a personal injury lien basis. This is essentially a promissory note that states if awards are received as a result of monies from a litigation lawsuit, then the medical fees will be paid out of the settlement reward.

The young man underwent the necessary surgery after much preparation. He did well afterwards and very slowly recovered to the point of being able to walk without a cane. As of the writing of this book, he still has not returned to soccer, as any type of running is too painful for him. It is yet to be determined whether he has ilioinguinal neuralgia or genital femoral neuralgia.

These are two conditions that may occur as a result of hernia repair. Occasionally, what happens during this procedure is that the mesh used as a fabric to repair the abdominal wall can sometimes trap nerves, which can grow into the mesh material. These nerves then send out abnormal pain signals, and the patient is left with a chronic pain syndrome. Diagnosis and treatment of this condition is paramount to the patient's recovery. It is yet to be determined if the aforementioned patient will develop one of these complications as a result of what would normally have been an uncomplicated hernia repair. Often, delay in surgery, as indicated in this instance, can predispose to a less than optimal surgical result. It is yet to be determined if such complications of surgery will be present.

Please refer to the website www.gotpaindocs.com, www.thegreatPainJack.com, or www.thegreatPainJack.org for further information.

Pelvic Pain Questionnaire–Answer these questions to map pain symptoms

*(Copy and fill out these worksheets and bring to your doctor. He/she may have his/her own, but answers to these questions provide a good overview of your pain condition and will help you develop a **pain profile** in order to use your time with your doctor more effectively.)*

Where is your pain located? _____

In what part of the pelvis does the pain seem to be most prominent? _____

Is it also in your abdomen /flanks /back? _____

When does your pain start and end? _____

Is it related to mealtime? _____ Sexual intercourse? _____

Does it occur one hour after eating? _____

When did you first begin to have pelvic pain, to the best of your recollection?

Where does your pelvic pain travel to? _____

Is it continuous throughout the day or associated with your period? _____

Has your pelvic pain ever improved? _____

Is it relieved with bowel movements? _____ Worse with intercourse? _____
_____

Has it become chronic? _____

Is it associated with nausea and vomiting? _____

Could there be two or more different types of pain syndromes that seem to occur simultaneously? _____

Does your pelvic pain wax and wane, or does it stay at the same intensity throughout the course of the day? _____

Does the pain occur all over your body as well as the pelvis? _____

Which pelvic pain bothers you the most? _____

Does eating or fasting help the pelvic pain get better? _____

Do you have a systemic disease diagnosed previously that may be contributing to your pelvic pain? _____

Perhaps celiac sprue? (gluten intolerance), or perhaps lactose intolerance? _____

Do you have a history of cancer of any abdominal or pelvic organs? _____

Have you had hepatitis before? _____

Do you have a history of heavy drinking? _____

Is there any history of bleeding from the gastrointestinal tract, including vomiting or spitting up dark blood? _____

Do you believe your pelvic pain is caused by accident or injury? _____

Could this pelvic pain have begun as a work-related injury? _____

Does your pelvic pain feel like a muscular ache? _____

Could an old injury that did not heal be exacerbated by current daily activities? _____
_____

Use the following scale to describe the severity of your pain for each type of pain you have, with one being the least amount of pain and 10 being the highest level of pain you could ever imagine: 1 ... 2 ... 3 ... 4 ... 5 ... 6 ... 7 ... 8 ... 9 ... 10.

What descriptors can you use for your pain: Burning? Aching? Shooting? Sharp? Throbbing? Cramping? Constant? Numbing? Lancinating? Stabbing? Transient? Excruciating? Tingling? On fire?

Does your pain get worse or better with sitting, bending, lifting, walking, grasping, sweeping, standing, crawling, squatting, reaching overhead, eating, coughing, sneezing, physical activity, stress, driving, sexual intercourse, heat, ice, physical therapy, medications? _____

Have any of the following treatments provided relief of your pain condition: Surgery? Medications? Injection therapy? Chiropractic? Tens unit (electric stimulation)? Physical therapy? Traction? Heat therapy? Bed rest? Acupuncture? Psychotherapy? _____
_____

Specific questions regarding pelvic pain to best allow you and your doctor to make a diagnosis

Does the pain seem to arise in the midpelvis or lower part of the pelvis? _____ Could it be referred to the pelvis? _____

Is the pelvic pain fleeting, transient, intermittent? Does it come in waves or cycles? Is the pain constant and/or throbbing? _____ Is the pain sharp?

Is the pelvic pain associated with a vascular phenomenon? Menstrual periods? Premenstrual syndrome? _____ Sexual function?

Is the pelvic pain associated with numbness or tingling? _____ Weakness of any of the muscles of the abdomen? _____ Paralysis? _____ Increased or decreased sweating? Skin discoloration? Skin rash anywhere on the body? Tingling pins and needles on the face or body? _____ Cold? _____ Muscle spasm tightness? _____ Trouble sleeping? "Touch me not" pain? _____

Is there a history of sexually transmitted disease or urologic dysfunction? _____

Is there a history of food allergies? _____ Is there a history of Crohn's disease or ulcerative colitis? _____

Is there a history of pancreatic disease or cancer? _____ Is there a history of diabetes? _____

What improves your pelvic pain? _____ What medications have you tried that failed? Have you had injections for your pelvic pain? _____ Celiac plexus nerve block? Pudendal or saddle block? _____ Other type of ilioinguinal, genitofemoral, iliohypogastric nerve block? Or other type of injection? _____-

What specifically helps your pelvic pain? Sleep? _____ Rest? Ice? _____ Heat? Pressure? Exercise? _____ Any type of therapy? _____ Any kind of surgery? _____ Have you used light or laser therapy to try to treat your abdominal pain? _____

What specific medications have you tried that failed? _____

What specific herbal or natural remedies have you tried? _____

Do you take supplements for your condition? _____

Is your pelvic pain accompanied with transient paralysis? _____ Do the muscles of your body go into spasm or become distorted at any time? _____ Do the abdominal/pelvic muscles appear to be weaker at any time? _____

Body Map for Pelvic Pain Questionnaire

Figure 8
Obstetric Pain

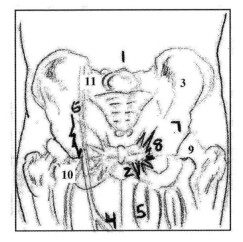

1. Pregnancy
2. Vulvodynia/Prostadynia
3. Gluteal Bursitis
4. Obturator Neuralgia
5. Adductor Tendonitis
6. Femoral Neuropathy
7. Psoas Bursitis
8. Osteitis Pubis
9. Piriformis Syndrome
10. Ischiogluteal Bursitis
11. Coccydynia

Figure 9

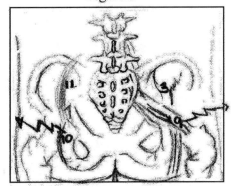

Figure 9
Back View/Obstetric Pain

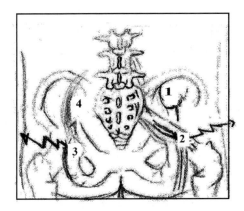

1. Gluteal Bursitis
2. Piriformis Syndrome
3. Ischiogluteal Bursitis
4. Coccydynia

Chapter 10

So, You've Got Neck Pain?

Case Study: *Mustafa came to my office looking dour. He had been plagued by neck pain for a good portion of his life. It all stemmed from a work-related injury that took place fifteen years earlier. He had worked as a mechanical contractor, a job which involved a lot of lifting over the head and shoulders, and had what appeared to be a simple cervical disc herniation.*

Y et it turned out to be much more complicated. Mustafa had undergone no less than eight cervical fusions and two low-back surgeries to stop his pain. Additional reconstructive neck surgeries left him with a painful postoperative condition. He sought solace in physical therapy and painkillers, whose dosage escalated over the years.

When I first saw Mustafa I noticed that his pain originated from postsurgical scar tissue in and around the neck nerves. I examined the area and found, to my horror, that the reconstructive neck surgery he had had done was a very old-fashioned procedure, classifiable by modern standards as essentially barbaric. The reconstruction involved a series of wires that were circumferentially threaded through the cervical vertebra. I had never seen anything like this in my twenty years of practice.

Mustafa said he had been to doctors all over California and elsewhere and was unimpressed with all of them. He believed that doctors "could not believe I was in that much pain or thought I was just plain faking it for financial gain. Yes, I was told that."

The only exception was his primary-care physician, who he considered excellent. "Returning from my first visit with Dr. P, my wife asked how it went. I told her that for the first time I feel like I found a doctor who appreciates my chronic condition, respects my pain, and treats me as a person instead of just another x-ray!

"Dr. P—— said I needed a new MRI. So I got one, and he reviewed it. He looked at me and said he believed I needed a total neck reconstruction, including the removal of the wires, pins, and adding rods in the back of my neck. He told me, 'This should eliminate the risk of paralysis during something like a slip and fall injury.'

"I couldn't believe my ears. I have been going to doctor after doctor, concerned about exactly *that, and none had listened to me. When I saw my neurosurgeon with a referral from Dr. P, he apologized for what the medical establishment had done to me. He said that no one should have had that many surgeries and asked if I was ready to end this travesty."*

Mustafa had the reconstructive neck surgery prescribed by Dr. P, but he developed an extremely painful condition afterward. My first instinct was to suppress the inflammation and irritation of the normal structures of the neck and spine, keeping in mind that the amount of radical surgery Mustafa had had would complicate any type of healing. My targeted injections would not be enough to put an end to all his pain.

I also noted that Mustafa had lost most of the function in his neck muscles. Was this a result of a loss of neurologic function or a muscle-wasting syndrome? One thing was clear: no one paid particular attention to the healing that would need to take place after his surgeries. No one prepared a rehabilitative plan for him.

I began to craft one. First, I modified the medications he was taking to stop the constant neck spasms he experienced and prescribed him painkillers for the pain coming from the nerves in the neck. Next, I ordered a series of steroid injections into the epidural space and nerve roots, which might have been prone to scarring. The response to the first set of injections was modest, at best.

We performed another procedure, known as a cervical facet injection, which blocks the sensory nerves in the joints in the back of the neck. This improved neck function and, more importantly, gave Mustafa hope that full relief was within reach.

Since we commonly measure pain on a scale of 1 to 10, 1 being the least amount of pain and 10 being the most, it was necessary to quantify Mustafa's relief after the recent procedures. After a few diagnostic and therapeutic injections, his pain moved down from 10 to 6. This was not good enough, but it marked significant progress. I assured him that we would not stop until we met our goal. I conferred with a number of neurosurgeons about the type of surgery he had previously undergone. The sentiment was that since he had significant surgery in the past without good results, he would not be a good candidate for additional surgery.

I contacted a well-respected, Stanford-trained spine surgeon who had rebuilt several spines the previous year with good results. I explained our predicament, vocalizing my concern that the old wires and reconstruction in Mustafa's 's neck were causing his pain. The neurosurgeon examined him and decided to remove all the remnants of the former surgeries, replacing them with new hardware.

I saw Mustafa after the surgery, and to say that he did not look good was an understatement. He had an excavation site in the back of his neck and spine that looked like a hand grenade blew off a chunk of his body. The massive muscle deficit was too tremendous to be filled. The surgery also robbed him of his ability to speak in a normal conversational tone, as some of the nerves controlling the ability to speak were cut during the surgery. He now communicated in an eerie, raspy whisper.

We engaged in intense postoperative therapy. I performed a series of muscular trigger-point injections and cervical facet joint blocks that, after ten weeks, brought down the severity of his pain to a modest 3 out of 10 during the day.

I brought in a neuromuscular chiropractic specialist, who analyzed Mustafa's posture and weakened neck musculature. He prescribed stretches, strengthening exercises, and active release techniques targeting his neck and back. His pain, with moderate medication and these exercises, seemed to reach a plateau of 3 or 4 out of 10.

Then something truly amazing happened. One day I was checking my e-mails, and, since it was around Easter, I stumbled upon a religious-themed, healing-type e-mail forwarded to me by someone. Quite accidentally, Mustafa's name popped up in my forward list, and I hit the send button without realizing it until after the fact.

About four weeks later, with the whole event out of my mind, Mustafa told me during a routine visit that he needed to speak to me personally. I let him in, and he closed the door after him. He had a stern look on his face. My heart pounded, and I felt the day's fatigue wearing down on me. He spoke in his usual raspy whisper.

He said that in the last few months he was having a difficult time with the fact that his condition, though significantly improved, had not been completely resolved. But then he thanked me for forwarding him the aforementioned e-mail. At first I didn't know what he was talking about, but then it hit me. Brian said that usually when he sits at the computer his back and neck pain flares up. However, when he opened the e-mail from me his pain was entirely gone.

He admitted he was not a religious person, but he believed that something miraculous had taken place. For the first time in over fifteen years, he had zero pain and was overjoyed. I shared in his joy. Whether it was a miracle, or a combination of luck, good medicine, and surgery, I truly think that if a person believes in his doctor's abilities and wishes to be healed, he or she can be healed. Nine months earlier we had embarked on a mission to heal Mustafa's condition, and I can say that mission has finally been accomplished.

Neck pain can result from injury or, seeing as the neck is one of the most important supporting structures in the body, simply from regular wear and tear stress. It can give rise to arm, shoulder, hand, and head pain, and it is responsible for hours of lost productivity and needless suffering. Please refer to the websites www.gotpaindocs.com, www.thegreatPainJack.com, or www.thegreatPainJack.org for further information.

Cervical Facet Syndrome

Cervical facet syndrome consists of neck pain, headaches, and shoulder pain. The pain can be dull, either one or two-sided, and it can increase by flexing or extending the neck or by bending from side to side. The pain is agitated by physical exercise. Often the patient will show decreased range of motion of the cervical spine.

Diagnosis and Treatment

X-ray examination of the cervical spine (especially after age fifty) will show some degree of arthritis or abnormality of the facet joints of the cervical spine. MRI and CT scans can be performed to determine whether arthritis within the facet joints contributes to the painful condition. Since other conditions, such as cervical fibromyositis, cervical bursitis, cervicalgia, inflammatory arthritis, and disorders of the cervical spinal cord can mimic cervical facet syndrome, the doctor may attempt an anesthetic injection into the suspect diseased facet joints to complete the diagnosis.

Case Study: I went to a local hospital to evaluate Mercedes, an eighty-two-year-old woman who had fallen while working in her rose garden. She had tripped over a brick and fallen right on her face. Though she was put on very strong painkillers such as morphine and Vicodin upon arrival at the hospital, she complained of extremely tender neck pain and difficulty with her back.

The doctors checked her for face, shoulder, neck, and back injuries. Various tests were performed, but she still needed a cervical MRI study to complete the assessment. When I arrived I ordered a lower-back study and the MRI, and the results came back relatively benign. Nevertheless, a colleague of mine indicated that she had fairly extensive facial bruising and extremely rigid neck movements. The physical therapist said the spasms in her neck were too extensive to even attempt physical therapy.

Mercedes had tender areas at the base of her skull, which pointed toward occipital neuralgia and cervical myospasm. She categorized the intensity of the pain as an 8 on a 10-point scale, and just one look at her confirmed that she was not exaggerating.

Although reluctant at first, she agreed to an occipital nerve block injection into her neck muscles. Five minutes after I administered the shot, she felt remarkably better. She said her pain had entirely disappeared.

I was happy that she was finally able to go home after over seven days at the hospital. Later, it turned out that her successful treatment was rewarding on another level: she was a hospital board member.

After an MRI confirms *a chronic* cervical facet syndrome, the condition may be treated through multiple options. Physical therapy, including heat and massage therapy, may be combined with nonsteroidal anti-inflammatory medication and muscle relaxants. Chiropractic therapy may also provide relief for a number of individuals. Cervical facet blocking injection is a reasonable approach if the above measures fail. If the pain relief from cervical facet blocks is short-lived, a procedure known as radiofrequency ablation can be performed for lasting duration. This involves burning nerves in the area using radiofrequency energy, thus eliminating the pain on a semipermanent basis.

Cervical Radiculopathy

Cervical radiculopathy consists of neck and upper extremity pain arising from the cervical nerve roots. This pain is usually accompanied by numbness, weakness, and loss of reflexes. The causes of cervical radiculopathy include herniated discs, arthritis, tumors, and infection. Patients with this condition may experience extreme weakness and a lack of coordination in the affected limb. Muscle spasms and neck pain, as well as pain in the muscles in the shoulders, are common. Cervical radiculopathy can lead to compression of the spinal cord, resulting in a condition known as myelopathy. Cervical myelopathy may include lower extremity weakness and bowel and bladder symptoms that can constitute a neurosurgical emergency.

Diagnosis and Treatment

Cervical radiculopathy can be best treated using conservative means. This will include physical therapy, heat packs, massages, nonsteroidal anti-inflammatory medication, and skeletal muscle relaxants. Chiropractic manipulation may help in the early stages to relieve pain in the arms and shoulders, as well as headaches. Cervical epidural injections with local anesthetics and steroids have been proven to be extremely effective in the treatment of cervical radiculopathy. If epidural steroid injections do not prove successful, cervical discography may be necessary to isolate a diseased disk. Such procedures may be performed with a mechanical decompression device or a device that uses radiofrequency energy to vaporize a small amount of nucleus of the disc known to be the problem. Please refer to the website www.gotpaindocs.com, www.thegreatPainJack.com, or www.thegreatPainJack.org for further information.

Case Study: I was summoned by the State of California to give a medical opinion on a middle-aged secretary, Mrs. E——, who worked for the sheriff's department. She had suffered from chronic headaches for over three years, and the headaches were usually attended by a severe, stabbing neck pain. She had already received injections of occipital nerve blocks into the base of her skull to alleviate her headaches. They helped for a few weeks, but then the pain returned, worse than before.

When I first met Mrs. E——, she told me that her former doctor performed a radiofrequency ablation, which relieved her neck pain but not the headaches. Due to the modest success of the procedure, her doctor requested the health insurance carrier's approval to perform it several more times. This of course raised a red flag for the health insurance company, especially since the doctor never tried basic cervical epidural steroid injections. As a result, the carrier denied all future care based on failure to demonstrate the benefit of the procedures already performed.

I asked E—— to describe her pain for me. She said she felt a constant, unrelenting, dull, stabbing pain in the back of her neck and scalp, which was accompanied by an excruciating, lancinating headache whenever she sat up.

I requested a weight-bearing MRI of E's neck to get a closer look. This test requires the patient to stand as it scans her neck in various flexed positions and is fairly controversial in the medical community. Most MRI studies are performed in the lying-down position; however, this does not reflect our true anatomical posture. Therefore, as some of the medical community believes, as in E's case, the additional cost and time associated with weight-bearing MRI studies are worth the extra effort to make the diagnosis.

Nevertheless, the carrier did not approve this diagnostic procedure. I was furious. I assaulted the carrier with calls and letters, demanding an approval, threatening penalties for denying a diagnostic test, which I equated with an obstruction of justice in a legal proceeding. I finally got the okay to move ahead with the weight-bearing MRI.

The results showed severe abnormalities in E's anatomy, including neural foraminal stenosis, disk protrusion with herniations, and an overgrown bony spring in her spine. These findings explained the headaches and lancinating neck pain she experienced.

It became obvious that she had not been diagnosed sooner because the results I discovered would not be detected by a regular MRI. It is also likely the abnormalities became worse as she continued working.

After submitting my report, Mrs. E—— was approved for the necessary medical treatment and thanked me effusively for helping her. I felt great joy in knowing that I had picked the proper fight with the insurance company and that it ultimately led to a proper diagnosis and resolution of her condition. Of course, the insurance company would have rather thrown out her case as phony and insubstantial, saving an inordinate amount of money, but that is why it is so important for doctors to fight for their patients.

Fibromyalgia of the Cervical Spine

Fibromyalgia of the cervical spine is one of the most common conditions in clinical practice. Fibromyalgia (discussed at greater length in another chapter of this book) is a chronic pain syndrome that affects a regional or global portion of the body. The diagnosis is made by examination and confirmation of tender points in certain known body regions. After proper diagnosis, treatment of fibromyalgia may include therapeutic application of heat and cold, and medications including muscle relaxants and antidepressants, as well as the use of a TENS unit (transcutaneous electrical nerve stimulation). Cervical epidural and BOTOX injections have also been used to treat this condition.

Cervical Strain

Cervical strain is a collection of symptoms that consists of nonparticular neck pain radiating into the shoulders. Headaches are commonplace, giving rise to emotional stress and sleep abnormalities. The *trapezius* muscle (located between the shoulder and base of the neck) usually undergoes spasms, limiting the range of motion of the top of the spine. Cervical strain results from trauma to the cervical spine.

Diagnosis and Treatment

A diagnosis includes finding tender or spasmodic neck muscles and a decreased range of motion in the neck. An MRI study should be performed if headache symptoms or pain at the base of the neck is persistent. Cervical strain may be confused with bursitis, cervical fibromyositis, inflammatory arthritis, and disorders of the cervical spinal cord, roots, plexus, and nerves.

Cervical strain can be treated with chiropractic therapy, heat and cold application, acupuncture, and massages. Medications, including anti-inflammatories and muscle relaxants, will help ease the aching nature of the pain. Cervical facet and cervical epidural steroid injections can also provide relief.

Brachial Plexus

Diseases of the brachial plexus, namely the collection of nerve trunks descending from the neck into the armpit, produce symptoms that affect the neck. Causes of brachial plexus disease include tumors, direct trauma to the plexus such as stretch injuries, and inflammations. Patients suffering from this disease complain of pain that has a boring, dull quality. Often movement of the neck and shoulders will worsen the pain.

Pancoast's Tumor Syndrome

Pancoast's tumor syndrome results from the growth of a tumor on the brachial plexus. Characteristics of this syndrome are severe arm pain, eye droop, and occasionally the tumor may grow so large as to crush the ribs. Occasionally patients with this condition will not move their shoulder at all for fear of developing intractable pain.

Treatment of this condition should be directed toward the type of cell that is detected in the tumor. Typical options are surgery, chemotherapy, and radiation. Medications such as opioid analgesics, or baclofen, an antiseizure drug, should be used to promote pain relief. A brachial plexus block can be performed with a local anesthetic and steroid injection, which will rapidly relieve pain. If the brachial plexus block is successful in reducing painful symptoms, the radiofrequency ablation technique discussed earlier can be used to destroy the nerve fibers of the brachial plexus.

Though rare, seatbelt injuries have been known to contribute to brachial plexus problems and can be treated with brachial plexus injections of anesthetic and steroid. Stretch injuries and contusions of the brachial plexus can be treated with similar strategies.

Please refer to the website www.gotpaindocs.com, www.thegreatPainJack.com, or www.thegreatPainJack.org for further information.

Thoracic Outlet Syndrome

This syndrome refers to a collection of signs and symptoms that include aching pain of the neck, arm, and shoulder, thought to result from the compression of the brachial plexus. This is more commonly noted in women of age groups twenty through fifty.

The so-called Adson test can determine if thoracic outlet syndrome is present. A confirmation will come in the form of a reduction in the patient's pulse rate in the affected side with the neck extended toward the affected side.

Generally speaking, physical therapy should be performed as a first-line treatment for brachial plexus syndrome. Medications including gabapentin, antiseizure medication, and muscle relaxants should be prescribed to reduce symptoms. A brachial plexus block with local anesthetic and steroid can complement the treatment of thoracic outlet syndrome.

Correct and prompt diagnosis is critical to the success of treating these conditions. Stretch injuries and contusions of the brachial plexus may respond to conservative care, but complications stemming from the invasion by tumor (like the aforementioned Pancoast's syndrome) will require aggressive surgical treatment. In either case, brachial plexus block represents a state-of-the-art interventional treatment option for these difficult-to-treat conditions.

> *Case Study: A young woman, Zoe, was referred to me for injuries sustained after a near head-on car collision. Despite several visits to a chiropractor, she complained of intractable headaches that occurred almost every day. Though there was no indication of head injury, whiplash in the neck was certain.*
>
> *An MRI study revealed discs that had small herniations, which were dismissed by her doctor and chiropractor. After a cervical epidural injection only modestly improved her headaches, I decided to test the herniated discs in her neck to see if they were responsible for her pain.*
>
> *The test known as discography involves placing a needle in the center of the disc and injecting it with a dye. The findings of the dye study are recorded using a flouroscope and are paired with an MRI and a CAT scan to verify the origin of the pain within the disc structures. Zoe had two discs in her neck that tested positive for symptomatic concordant pain and were responsible for inducing her headaches. These discs were treated with a radiofrequency ablation device that vaporized a small portion of the affected discs. Zoe's 's headaches stopped immediately. Please refer to the website www.gotpaindocs.com or search you tube .com at channel drjohnpetrgalia or the pain doctors for further information.*

Neck Pain Questionnaire–Answer these questions to map pain symptoms

*(Copy and fill out these worksheets and bring to your doctor. He/she may have his/her own, but answers to these questions provide a good overview of your pain condition and will help you remember and collect a **pain profile** in order to use your time with your doctor more effectively.)*

Where is your pain located?

When does your pain start and end?

When did you first begin to have pain, to the best of your recollection?

Where does your pain travel to?

Is it continuous throughout the day?

Has your pain ever improved?

Has it become chronic?

Are there two or more different types of pain syndromes that seem to occur simultaneously?

Does your pain wax and wane, or does it stay at the same intensity throughout the course of the day?

Does the pain occur all over?

Which pain bothers you the most?

Do the different pains that you have come from different areas and appear to be related to different conditions or movements of the face or body?

Which pain would you like to get rid of the most?

Do you have a systemic disease diagnosed previously that may be contributing to your pain?

Do you believe your pain is caused by accident or injury?

Was this a work-related injury?

Could an old injury that did not heal be exacerbated by current daily activities?

Use the following scale to describe the severity of your pain for each type of pain you have,

with one being the least amount of pain and 10 being the highest level of pain you could ever imagine: 1 … 2 … 3 … 4 … 5 … 6 … 7 … 8 … 9 … 10.

What descriptors can you use for your pain: Burning? Aching? Shooting? Sharp? Throbbing? Cramping? Constant? Numbing? Lancinating? Stabbing? Transient? Excruciating? Tingling? On fire?

Does your pain get worse or better with sitting, bending, lifting, walking, grasping, sweeping, standing, crawling, squatting, reaching overhead, eating, coughing, sneezing, physical activity, stress, driving, sexual intercourse, heat, ice, physical therapy, medications?

Have any of the following treatments provided relief of your pain condition: Surgery? Medications? Injection therapy? Chiropractic? Tens unit (electric stimulation)? Physical therapy? Traction? Heat therapy? Bed rest? Acupuncture? Psychotherapy?

Specific questions regarding neck pain to best help you and your doctor to make an accurate diagnosis

Does the neck pain seem to arise in the neck region or does it appear to come from another area that can be directed to the neck? _____

Is the neck pain fleeting, transient, or constant and throbbing? _____

Does the neck pain radiate down the arms? _____

If you have had extensive dental work, do you still have pain coming from the teeth? _____ Have you had extensive dental extractions? _____

Is the neck pain associated with: Numbness? Weakness? Paralysis? _____ Increased or decreased sweating? Skin discoloration? Skin rash anywhere on the face or body? Tingling pins and needles on the neck or body? _____ Cold? _____ Muscle spasm? Tightness? _____ Trouble sleeping? "Touch me not" pain? _____

What improves your neck pain? _____ What medications have you tried that failed? Have you had injections for your pain? _____ Do any of these modalities helped your neck pain: Sleep? _____ Rest? Ice? _____ Heat? Pressure? Exercise? _____ Any type of therapy? _____ Any kind of surgery? _____ Have you used light or laser therapy to try to treat your neck pain? Do you use any rubs or topical agents to treat your neck pain? _____

What specific medications have you tried that failed? _____

What specific herbal or natural remedies have you tried? _____

Do you take supplements for your condition? _____

Is your neck pain accompanied with headaches? _____ How would you best describe these headaches? _____

Is your pain accompanied with transient paralysis? _____ Do the muscles of your face or neck go into spasm or become distorted at any time? _____ Do the expressions of the facial or neck muscles appear to be weaker at any time? _____ Do the neck muscles or the ability to hold the head in position fail or tire easily? _____

Body Map for Neck Pain Questionnaire

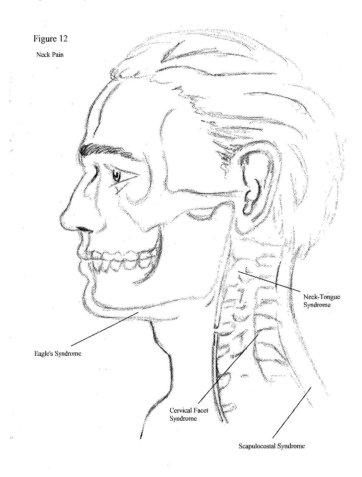

Figure 12

Neck Pain

Neck-Tongue
Syndrome

Eagle's Syndrome

Cervical Facet
Syndrome

Scapulocostal Syndrome

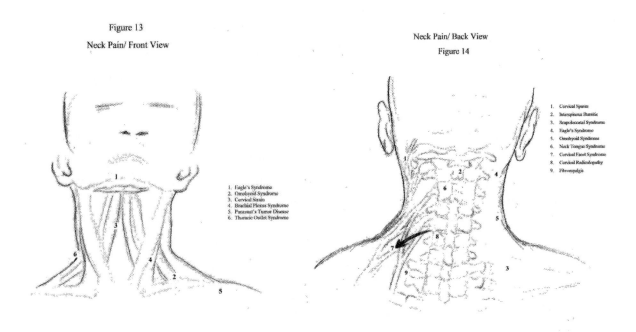

Figure 13

Neck Pain/ Front View

1. Eagle's Syndrome
2. Omohyoid Syndrome
3. Cervical Strain
4. Brachial Plexus Syndrome
5. Pancoast's Tumor Disease
6. Thoracic Outlet Syndrome

Neck Pain/ Back View

Figure 14

1. Cervical Spasm
2. Interspinous Bursitis
3. Scapulocostal Syndrome
4. Eagle's Syndrome
5. Omohyoid Syndrome
6. Neck Tongue Syndrome
7. Cervical Facet Syndrome
8. Cervical Radiculopathy
9. Fibromyalgia

Chapter 11:

So, You've Got Back Pain?

Case Study: *A woman in her forties, Ms. D——, came to my office with a history of back pain. English was not her first language, and she had trouble communicating what was bothering her. Her husband, who accompanied her, did most of the talking for her.*

She had had a vague back pain for some time, and her lower as well as occasionally upper extremities would feel weak. Neither a physical exam nor an MRI shed light on this weakness. Fortunately, I had copies of her lab results from a recent trip to the hospital for a steroid injection to treat degenerative lumbar disc disease. These studies including an EKG, serum electrolytes, glucose, a blood count, and a chest x-ray. After this routine injection, D—— was admitted to the recovery area. That's when she began to exhibit very odd symptoms.

She said she felt extremely weak and could not hold up her hands or neck on her own. And yet, after examining her, I found no specific motor or sensory block that could account for her condition.

Worse, Mrs. D—— informed me that she was having some difficulty breathing, her large frame sagging and looking very fatigued. At the same time, she asked for a soft drink, baffling me and the nurses. It seemed unlikely that anyone with breathing problems, experiencing a neurological dysfunction of some kind, would ask for a soft drink.

I ordered an oxygen mask for her and listened to her lungs, which sounded clear. Yet she was growing weaker, and I began to worry about her going into respiratory arrest. I had another round of laboratory studies done, along with an emergency lumbar MRI study.

My thoughts rapidly turned toward possible causes for her condition, a list extending before my eyes: inadvertent puncture of the cerebral spinal fluid; stroke; transient ischemic attack; epidural hematoma; uncontrolled bleeding around the spine, causing sudden neurological dysfunction; low blood glucose; high blood glucose; Guillian-Barre syndrome, which causes transient or permanent motor and sensory weakness; multiple sclerosis; and electrolyte abnormalities.

It was now seven o'clock at night, and Mrs. D—— would have normally been discharged four hours ago. The new MRI study came back looking exactly like the preceding one. This at least eliminated the possibility of epidural hematoma. I reviewed her history with her *husband and focused on the only two other times that she had such nearly paralyzing attacks of weakness. I pressed him for details regarding these events, but he did not offer any new useful information.*

I looked over the tests again. Initial lab studies done the morning of D's admission to the hospital indicated completely normal serum electrolyte levels. Electrolytes are essential ingredients, including sodium, potassium, chloride, bicarbonate, and glucose, in the plasma of our blood that keep us functioning normally. Even small changes in their composition can affect neurological, cognitive, and skeletal/muscular function. I compared her morning results with those after the injections and found a drop in the serum potassium levels from 4.2 mcg down to 2.1 mcg per deciliter.

Suddenly it hit me, in the strangest form. I remembered a video I saw many, many years ago of a dog that had a condition known as hypokalemia periodic paralysis. *The dog, trained to catch a flying disk would, under certain conditions, literally become paralyzed almost in midair. The reason for the paralysis was a pathologic inability to maintain a normal serum potassium level. Could D, who had already suffered two nearly fatal attacks of respiratory paralysis, have hypokalemia periodic paralysis?*

This was the only theory that made sense to me at this point. I immediately requested a potassium supplement to her regular IV fluids. Shortly, her condition began to improve, and she was finally able to leave the hospital about nine o'clock that evening. When I explained how I made the diagnosis of this relatively rare condition, she seemed relieved to know there was an explanation for her weakness.

Later, I realized that the administration of the steroid pushed the serum potassium to a critical level in the blood. Since Mrs. D——'s body could not adapt quickly to low serum potassium levels, intravenous fluids with potassium administration, respiratory support with oxygen, and tincture of time had to preserve her vital neurological and respiratory functions.

Since formulating my diagnosis, Mrs. D—— has been referred to an endocrinologist. I saw her again a few months later, and her back pain was entirely gone.

The major cause of back pain is poor posture, which causes pain in the back muscles. Of course there are other conditions that may predispose someone to experience early and frequent back pain. Conditions such as rheumatoid, osteoarthritis, scoliosis, ankylosing spondylitis, and degenerative and traumatic disc disease cause back pain by affecting the spine. I will address these more common back pain causes in this chapter.

Over the course of human evolution the back, with its complex spine, has transformed from supporting quadrupeds, to us, upright bipeds. The anatomy of the spine is an amazingly complex living system, which can undergo growth and repair and which supports and maintains the brain and spinal cord.

The spinal cord and its connecting pairs of spinal nerves coordinate and provide motor and sensory function throughout your body. The spinal nerves exit from the spinal column through the *neuroforamina*, Latin for "window to the nerve." Separating the bones of the spinal column are disks, which are tough substances that give support between the bones of the spine. These discs are typically healthy, viable, and living tissue. A disk, however, is prone to rupture, herniation, or bulging under different types of stress. When it ruptures, the inner jelly-like material known as the *nucleus pulposus* may spill onto a nerve root. This is known as *disc herniation*.

> **Case Study:** *It was early in the morning, and I had just arrived at my Central Valley clinic. I entered through the waiting room and was immediately hit by a strong, foul smell. I asked one of my staff to put some fresh-cut, scented flowers in the holding area to neutralize the air as I moved on to my morning appointment.*
>
> *As I got closer to the examination room, I noticed that the smell grew stronger. When I opened the door I found a fifty-something-year-old man. Dirty, wearing scraps for clothes, his teeth virtually nonexistent, it must have been over a week since the last time he had bathed or changed clothes.*
>
> *He was covered in pus-filled lesions surely contributing to the smell he was exuding; they looked like Staphylococcus abscesses, and they were spread all over his arms and legs.*
>
> *The man was incommunicative and practically illiterate. When I asked him some basic questions about what day it was, or where he was, he could not give me a precise answer. After several attempts, he got the month right. I summoned his wife, who had equally poor hygiene and difficulty communicating. I wanted to establish why he was seeking care at a pain clinic, instead of at a hospital. It looked like he had signs of a wound infection at the site of what later turned out to be a neck surgery.*
>
> *I needed to figure out whether his abscesses or infection from this site were contributing to his mental confusion or whether the patient was mentally challenged. It seemed possible that an insidious infection had crept into his central nervous system, rendering his brain incapable of functioning correctly. However, seeing how there was no sign of fever or meningitis, I attributed mental slowness to illiteracy.*
>
> *I learned from his wife that he had worked as a landscaper and had suffered a work-related injury. I pressed her for details on the surgery, and she said that it was performed approximately three weeks ago. Afterwards, the surgeon placed her husband on antibiotics. She added that ten days later he "jumped off" a large truck and suffered disc injuries to his spine. This also apparently occurred on the job but was never accepted as a work-related claim. I suspected he had trouble communicating the severity of his pain to his employer.*
>
> *Piecing his medical history together proved quite difficult. My clinic usually asks for medical records and for any x-rays or MRI studies that may have been done on the patient prior to admittance. But all I got for this patient were some very poor, incomplete notes. Since he was on antibiotics for his neck, I focused on the rest of his body.*

What struck me as very odd was that the patient posed a large surgical risk: he was smoking one to two packs a day before and after his recent neck surgery. This not only undermined the potential success of the operation but also put him at risk of other conditions, such as a stroke, a heart attack, lung disease, etc. It also increases the likelihood of wound infection. For all of these reasons, many surgeons will not operate on patients if they are actively smoking during the preoperative period.

Why was surgery performed in the first place? I reviewed his MRI studies, which came to the clinic, and noticed that he had a cervical disc herniation that affected his cervical spinal cord. It had been there for over a year and a half and was incrementally growing more complex and dangerous. I understood now that the surgeon who operated on him had had a difficult choice to make between letting the condition spiral out of control and operating on someone who was a surgery risk.

I advised the patient to quit smoking immediately. Sometimes, with mentally-challenged patients, it is necessary to be very direct, and I was. I told him that if the infection worsened, he could die a painful, horrible death. I asked him if he had grandchildren. He did. I asked how many, and he said two. I asked them if he wanted to see them grow up, and he nodded. I told him they would not see him very long unless he quit smoking and treated his very serious wound infection with ultimate respect. He seemed to understand.

I decided he should continue taking his antibiotics. I have asked him to improve his personal hygiene and have prescribed him some analgesics for the pain. To this day he has serious back pain with multiple levels of degenerative discs and spine problems. This simple man nearly broke his back working hard, and he will probably not enjoy a healthy retirement.

We are still actively treating him, but we are waiting to implement treatment for his back until his wound heals. However, on the plus side, we won one small battle—he has quit smoking.

Lumbar Radiculopathy

Lumbar radiculopathy is a constellation of symptoms consisting of back and lower extremity pain arising from the lumbar nerve roots. In addition to pain, sufferers experience weakness, numbness, loss of reflexes, and tingling in the legs. The causes for lumbar radiculopathy include a herniated lumbar disc, blockage at the nerve root outlet, tumors, arthritic formation, and infection.

Occasionally a person who suffers from this condition will undergo a compression of the lumbar spinal nerve roots, which results in *lumbar myelopathy*. Patients suffering from this syndrome will experience lower extremity weakness and bowel and bladder symptoms. When this happens, it can constitute a serious emergency, and it usually is a good time to contact your local neurosurgeon.

Diagnosis and Treatment

MRI will provide information regarding the lumbar spine and its contents, and a CT scan may be used to detect any additional abnormalities. Studies known as electromyogram and nerve conduction velocity tests can be performed to diagnose the status of each individual nerve root in the lumbar plexus.

Treatment involves physical therapy with heat modalities, deep tissue massage combined with muscle relaxants, and nonsteroidal anti-inflammatory medication. Epidural lumbar steroid nerve blocks are a reasonable next step. For large disk herniations, disk decompression may be performed with needle-based techniques.

These techniques include inserting a needle into the center of the disc and chemically altering the damaged contents of the diseased disc with radiofrequency energy. This will promote the healthy regeneration of the disc and complete the healing process. Since sleep problems and depression may accompany lumbar radiculopathy, sleeping and antidepressant medication may be prescribed.

Case Study: Garret was a mess. He was in his late fifties; he was a veteran who had posttraumatic stress disorder, degenerative disc disease resulting from a failed back surgery, and spinal arthritis, which had been bothering him for over five years.

I found that injection therapy brought him the most relief, so I focused on fixing his back surgery with an implantable neurostimulator device. Basically, I surgically placed neurostimulator leads into his body. These leads would then produce a volley of current that would distract the brain and spinal cord from pain signals. This definitely reduced the severity of the pain he experienced.

A few years after the procedure, Garrett was involved in a big car accident. His wife, who was in the car with him, was left essentially disabled. She lost her job. Garrett also had a few grandchildren, who all moved back into his house for a variety of reasons. His children were unemployed. He too became unable to work because of his pain.

The pleasure he got from riding his Harley came to an abrupt end. Soon his financial situation began to collapse. He had to choose between losing his house or selling his motorcycle. His back pain caused him to take more painkillers. All the progress we had made managing his pain over the years had literally dissolved in front of our eyes. It got worse.

One day my office manager came to me and told me that her car license tag was gone. It was there when she arrived and was gone when she checked in the evening before leaving work. She thought that maybe since the new tag had been recently applied it may have just fallen off. Dismayed and confused by this information, I decided to check our video surveillance footage from the last few days.

There it was. A grainy video showed Garrett slinking around the parking lot to my office manager's car and removing the license tag. I could not believe what I saw. We had been treating him for over five years, often without any payment. Why would he suddenly steal from us?

I had to dismiss Garrett from our practice. I referred him to three other pain clinics in the area. But none of them would admit him, and the only one that considered it had a six-week waiting period. I feared that he might go into withdrawal if he had to wait six weeks, but I could not accept him.

He would call our clinic to apologize, asking to speak to me directly. I never took his calls, though, and stood firm by my decision.

One day, Garrett arrived at the clinic looking utterly defeated. He refused to leave unless he could speak to me. Though wary, I agreed to speak to him privately. Garrett told me that he had to sell his Harleys. However, in order to do so, he would have to put it in the local dealer showroom. He found out that the store did not take consignment items without current registration and a proof of insurance. He said he spent the $350 on insurance, but he could not afford the registration fees. Since his financial situation was dire, he was forced to make a decision. He was desperate to get the motorcycles listed. And it was in this desperation that he stole my office manager's registration tag.

He grew tearful as he spoke. He began apologizing profusely and begged for forgiveness and a reacceptance into the clinic. I looked at him and told him to wait. I went outside and asked my entire staff to enter the room. He then asked each of them for forgiveness. I asked if they were able to accept his apologies. I told them and him that I accepted them. The rest of the staff followed suit. And so Garrett, a veteran, was readmitted into our clinic on Veterans Day.

Spinal Stenosis

Spinal stenosis is the result of a narrowing of the spinal canal where the spinal cord lives. Pain and weakness in the legs and calves when walking, lying down, or standing accompany this condition. Spinal stenosis patients may also feel numbness and loss of reflexes in the lower extremities. The causes of spinal stenosis may be related to disc herniation, arthritis, and thickening of the supporting ligaments.

Fatigue and pain will improve if the patient flexes at the pelvis and assumes a sitting position. Extension of the spine may cause a flare-up in symptoms. Patients may complain of pain, tingling, and paresthesias in the affected nerve roots. There may be a lack of coordination in the affected extremity accompanied by muscle spasms and back pain transferred all the way into the shoulder.

Diagnosis and Treatment

Occasionally, spinal stenosis patients will undergo a compression of the lumbar spinal nerve roots, resulting in myelopathy, mentioned above. This will require emergency decompressive lumbar surgery. Prior to this, spinal decompression techniques such as "Radiofrequency energy or mechanical decompression" may be utilized. MRI of the lumbar spine as well as a CT scan is an excellent study to help make a diagnosis.

Treatment includes physical therapy, chiropractic, massage, nonsteroidal anti-inflammatory medications, and muscle relaxants. Lumbar or caudal epidural steroid nerve blocks may improve symptoms significantly. Please refer to the website www.gotpaindocs.com for further information.

Arachnoiditis

Arachnoiditis is not a fear of or inflammation due to spiders! It is a term used to describe thickening, scarring or inflammation of the arachnoid membrane, namely an outer cover of the lumbar nerve roots. The cause of this condition is unclear but is often attributed to herniated discs, infection, tumors, previous spine surgery, and spinal administration of medication. In addition to pain, arachnoiditis sufferers experience numbness, weakness, loss of reflexes, and bowel and bladder incontinence Muscle spasms and pain in the buttocks are typical. Like lumbar radiculopathy and spinal stenosis, arachnoiditis sufferers can experience compression of the lumbar spinal cord, resulting in myelopathy.

Diagnosis and Treatment

As with the conditions mentioned earlier, MRI and CT studies are necessary to help make the diagnosis. Treating arachnoiditis may be extremely difficult. Most efforts are geared toward decompressing the lumbar nerve roots and the spinal cord by treating the inflammatory component of the disease. This can be achieved with the administration of steroids, though sometimes surgery may be required. Antineuropathic agents such as *neurontin* may help diminish the symptoms.

Sacroiliac Joint Pain

Pain emanating from the sacroiliac joint comes when the patient lifts an object while in an awkward position. It is constant and is described as "speaking" in nature. The pain is localized around the sacroiliac joint, which is tender to the touch, and the upper leg, radiating into the buttocks and back of the legs. It never travels below the knees, though. Since activities such as walking aggravate the pain, rest can provide a relief of the symptoms.

Often the afflicted individual will favor the affected leg by tending to lean on the unaffected side. Spasms of the back muscles are common, and the range of motion in the lumbar spine in the upright position is limited. The pain usually improves when the sufferer sits.

The sacroiliac joint is susceptible to various types of arthritis, the most common of which is osteoarthritis. Sacroiliac joint pain can also result from collagen vascular diseases, infection, and Lyme disease. However, collagen vascular diseases usually cause pain in several joints, not just the sacroiliac joint. One of these diseases, *ankylosing spondylitis*, responds extremely well to injections of anesthetics and steroids.

Diagnosis and Treatment

X-rays and MRIs should be performed to confirm a diagnosis. Pain originating from the sacroiliac joint can be confused with lower back strain, lumbar bursitis, font arthritis, and diseases of the lumbar spinal cord, roots, plexus, and nerves. A physician may order bone scans to check for tumors and fractures that can be missed by an x-ray.

Initial treatment for this condition should include nonsteroidal anti-inflammatory medication and physical therapy. Chiropractic, acupuncture, and local application of heat alternated with cold may be beneficial in reducing symptoms as well. For symptoms that do not improve, injections of nerve blocks can produce remarkable results. If the injections are successful, radiofrequency lesioning may be carried out to burn nerves that line the sacroiliac joint. This may provide months of pain relief. Disorders of the sacroiliac joint are distinguishable from lumbar spine pain in that with the former condition one can bend forward. With lumbar spinal pain, on the other hand, this will aggravate the condition.

Piriformis Syndrome

This syndrome results from an entrapment of the sciatic nerve, which stretches from the lower back, through the buttock, to the legs. It has the distinction of being the longest nerve in the body. Piriformis syndrome is caused when the sciatic nerve is compressed by the piriformis muscle, whose primary function is to rotate the femur, i.e., the large bone of the thigh, outward, at the hip joint.

The resulting severe pain radiates from the buttocks into the legs and feet. Patients suffering from this condition may develop an abnormal gait, which can lead to other problems, such as back and hip pain. If untreated, the condition can lead to increasingly limited mobility of the legs.

Piriformis syndrome can be brought on by direct trauma, such as repetitive hip and lower extremity motions, or by repeated pressure on the piriformis muscle and the sciatic nerve.

Diagnosis and Treatment

Sufferers of piriformis syndrome experience tenderness in the affected area and occasionally an electric shock feeling upon contact. To make a diagnosis, your doctor may have you lie down and lift your leg straight up. If this test causes you pain, it is often a sign of sciatic nerve entrapment. Lifting or bending at the waist and hips, increases the pain in people suffering with piriformis syndrome. If untreated, the condition can cause a weakness and a wasting away of muscles in the lower extremities. The electromyogram test and x-rays of the back hip and pelvis can confirm the diagnosis.

Piriformis syndrome is often misdiagnosed as lumbar radiculopathy or is attributed to intra-articular hip disease. However, most patients suffering from a lumbar radiculopathy will have back pain associated with reflex, motor, and sensory changes, whereas piriformis syndrome will not affect a patient's reflexes. The motor and sensory changes are only limited to the sciatic nerve below the sciatic notch.

Treatment of pain and disability associated with piriformis syndrome should include a combination of nonsteroidal inflammatory medication and physical therapy. Repetitive activities that can exacerbate the symptoms should be avoided. During sleep, a pillow can be placed between the legs to ease the pain. Antineuropathic agents such as gabapentin (Neurontin) and pregabalain (Lyrica) may also decrease the nerve pain symptoms. Finally, an injection of a local anesthetic in combination with a steroid in the area of the sciatic nerve may alleviate some of the severe pain. In rare occasions, a surgical release of the sciatic nerve may be required. Please refer to the website www.gotpaindocs.com for further information.

Case Study: I once treated Rosa, a laundry woman, for a work-related injury involving persistent back and leg pain. She was sent to me by the state to do a Qualified Medical Evaluation to determine workers' compensation. Her former physician found nothing more than lumbar radiculopathy and strain, which he treated with rest and medication. However, the patient's condition did not improve after nine months of this minimal, conservative treatment. I ordered an MRI to see why the back pain had not improved, and the test came back completely normal.

Soon, it became clear to me that her former doctor misdiagnosed Rosa. She was actually suffering from piriformis syndrome. The laundry worker was then correctly treated for piriformis syndrome and sciatic nerve entrapment. Unfortunately, she had already developed a secondary gait abnormality and weakness of the affected muscles. Nevertheless, her integrity was preserved, and disability payments were recouped via a qualifying medical exam, proving that doctors do not always make the right diagnosis.

Case Study: A thirty-five-year-old man, Geoff, who had lost a lot of weight, complained to his family doctor of difficulty performing simple tasks due to back pain. The doctor recommended anti-inflammatory medications. His pain increased over the course of subsequent visits, and he began to seek the advice of other physicians to see what was causing his back pain.

X-rays revealed no specific abnormalities at first glance. Further, a surgeon told him he found nothing out of the ordinary. Soon, Geoff developed a reputation around doctors' offices as a person exaggerating his symptoms. Yet his pain refused to yield.

His family doctor ordered another set of x-rays of his lower back, which again returned inconclusive. As G's complaints continued, the doctor ordered a CAT scan of his spine. This revealed some very subtle bony abnormalities, known as a "pars defect." The pars is a part of the vertebrae that separates the facet joint from the rest of the vertebral bone.

When I met Geoff, I performed a standard lumbar epidural steroid injection, but it did not relieve his pain. Puzzled, I decided to see if the pars defect was the cause of the pain. My plan was to specifically inject the pars and see if the pain disappeared. Under local anesthesia, I injected the bony defect.

In the next fifteen minutes it became clear that we had nailed down the diagnosis. While during the injection Geoff writhed in pain, his symptoms nearly doubling, after a short while his pain dissipated, and his condition improved. Thus, despite previous misdiagnosis and accusations of fabrication of symptoms, we had discovered a very small area that caused immense problems for this otherwise healthy man.

I subsequently referred Geoff for orthopedic surgery by a trusted colleague. We then ran into another problem. Geoff's health insurance was extremely limited in its coverage. After dozens of calls, presentations, and arguments we finally obtained approval for the necessary surgery. Good thing, too, because it brought about the complete relief of his lower back pain.

Back Pain Questionnaire–Answer these questions to map pain symptoms

*(Copy and fill out these worksheets and bring to your doctor. He/she may have his/her own, but answers to these questions provide a good overview of your pain condition and will help you remember and collect a **pain profile** in order to use your time with your doctor more effectively.)*

Where is your pain located? _____

When does your pain start and end? _____

When did you first begin to have pain, to the best of your recollection?

Where does your pain travel to?

Is it continuous throughout the day?

Has your pain ever improved?

Has it become chronic?

Are there two or more different types of pain syndromes that seem to occur simultaneously?

Does your pain wax and wane, or does it stay at the same intensity throughout the course of the day?

Does the pain occur all over?

Which pain bothers you the most?

Do the different pains that you have come from different areas and appear to be related to different conditions or movements of the face or body?

Which pain would you like to get rid of the most?

Do you have a systemic disease diagnosed previously that may be contributing to your pain?

Do you believe your pain is caused by accident or injury?

Was this a work-related injury?

Could an old injury that did not heal be exacerbated by current daily activities?

Use the following scale to describe the severity of your pain for each type of pain you have,

with one being the least amount of pain and 10 being the highest level of pain you could ever imagine: 1 ... 2 ... 3 ... 4 ... 5 ... 6 ... 7 ... 8 ... 9 ... 10.

What descriptors can you use for your pain: Burning? Aching? Shooting? Sharp? Throbbing? Cramping? Constant? Numbing? Lancinating? Stabbing? Transient? Excruciating? Tingling? On fire?

9. Does your pain get worse or better with sitting, bending, lifting, walking, grasping, sweeping, standing, crawling, squatting, reaching overhead, eating, coughing, sneezing, physical activity, stress, driving, sexual intercourse, heat, ice, physical therapy, medications?

Have any of the following treatments provided relief of your pain condition: Surgery? Medications? Injection therapy? Chiropractic? Tens unit (electric stimulation)? Physical therapy? Traction? Heat therapy? Bed rest? Acupuncture? Psychotherapy?

Specific questions regarding back pain to help you and your doctor make an accurate diagnosis

Does the back pain seem to arise in the back region primarily, or does it appear to come from another area that can be directed to the lower back? _____

Is the lower back pain fleeting, transient, or constant and throbbing? _____

Does the lower back pain radiate down one or both legs? _____

If you have had back surgery, do you still have pain coming from the same area? _____ A different area? _____

Is the lower back pain associated with numbness? Weakness? Paralysis? _____ Increased or decreased sweating? Skin discoloration? Skin rash anywhere on the face or body? Tingling pins and needles on the neck or body? _____ Cold? _____ Muscle spasm? Tightness? _____ Trouble sleeping? "Touch me not" pain? _____

What improves your lower back pain? _____ What medications have you tried that failed? Have you had injections for your pain? _____ Have any of these modalities helped the lower back pain: Sleep? _____ Rest? Ice? _____ Heat? Pressure? Exercise? _____ Any type of therapy? _____ Any kind of surgery? _____ Have you used light or laser therapy to try to treat your back pain? _____ Do you use any rubs or topical agents to treat your back pain? _____

What specific medications have you tried that failed? _____

What specific herbal or natural remedies have you tried? _____

Do you take supplements for your condition? _____

Is your lower back pain accompanied with headaches? _____ How would you best describe these headaches? _____

Is your pain accompanied with transient paralysis? _____ Do the muscles of your lower back go into spasm or become distorted at any time? _____ Do the lower back muscles appear to be weaker at any time? _____ Do the lower back muscles or the ability to hold the spine in position fail or tire easily? _____

Body Map for Back Pain Questionnaire

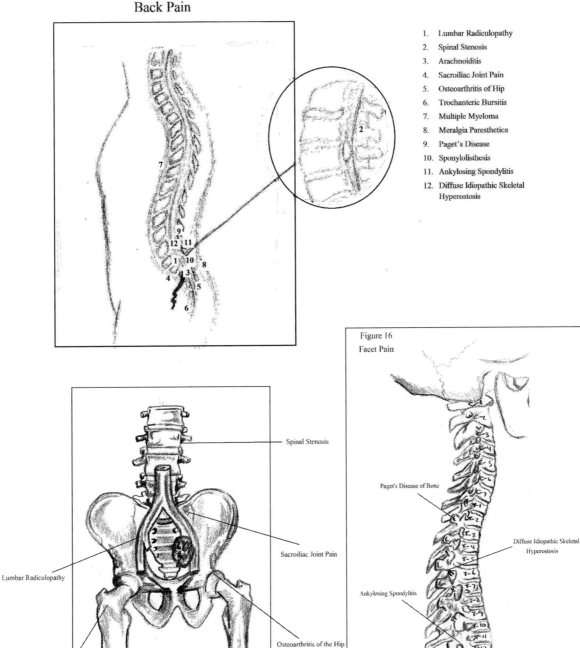

Figure 17
Back Pain

1. Lumbar Radiculopathy
2. Spinal Stenosis
3. Arachnoiditis
4. Sacroiliac Joint Pain
5. Osteoarthritis of Hip
6. Trochanteric Bursitis
7. Multiple Myeloma
8. Meralgia Paresthetica
9. Paget's Disease
10. Sponylolisthesis
11. Ankylosing Spondylitis
12. Diffuse Idiopathic Skeletal Hyperostosis

Figure 16
Facet Pain

Spinal Stenosis

Paget's Disease of Bone

Diffuse Idiopathic Skeletal Hyperostosis

Sacroiliac Joint Pain

Ankylosing Spondylitis

Lumbar Radiculopathy

Osteoarthritis of the Hip

Trochanteric Bursitis

Sponylolisthesis

Figure 15
Back Pain

Chapter 12

So, You've Got Knee Pain?

Case Study: I once treated a cage fighter Alfonso, who had multiple surgeries on his knees for instability and pain. After his second reconstructive surgery, he still complained of pain in his knee. His surgeon told him there was nothing more that could be done for him. His cage-fighting days were definitely over.

I wasn't so sure about this pronouncement. I began a series of diagnostic injections only and discovered the reason for his pain. Alfonso suffered from a combination of medial collateral ligament syndrome and suprapatella bursitis. With injections and physical therapy, his knee was fully rehabilitated, and the patient was able to return to his cage.

Arthritis of the knee, one of the most common causes of knee pain, is very painful and can damage the cartilage in the joint. Osteoarthritis is the most common form of arthritis resulting in knee pain, with posttraumatic and rheumatoid arthritis being a close second. Other causes of knee pain include infection, collagen vascular diseases, nodular synovitis, and Lyme disease.

Arthritis

Acute infectious arthritis is usually accompanied by fever and malaise. Collagen vascular diseases will generally affect multiple joints as opposed to being limited to the knee. Knee pain secondary to arthritis is localized around the knee and the distal femur, namely the long bone in the upper thigh. The pain is constant and throbbing in nature, interfering with sleep and limiting the patient's range of motion. Sometimes, a patient will experience a grating or popping sensation, known as *crepitus*. Activity will aggravate the condition, and advanced arthritis can lead to muscle atrophy and frozen knee.

Diagnosis and Treatment

X-rays are the best test to determine if you have arthritic knee pain. A complete blood count sedimentation rate can indicate if arthritis affects more than just one knee. Occasionally, disc disease with lumbar radiculopathy may mimic the pain associated with arthritis.

Similarly, bursitis of the knee may coexist with arthritis. Though rare, a tumor of the femur may appear to be related to knee arthritis.

Initial treatment of pain associated with arthritis should include nonsteroidal anti-inflammatory medications, physical therapy, and the application of heat and cold. Injections of a local anesthetic and a steroid are the next step in treating moderate to severe knee arthritis. Following such an injection, the relief is usually immediate.

> **Case Study:** *I was once visited by a professional skateboarder, Cody, age twenty-three, who came into the office limping. He complained of knee and occasional back pain. He said that his career heavily depended on his knees, which, he felt, were shot. Reluctantly, he faced the threat of early retirement due to several skateboarding injuries.*

I reviewed his x-rays, which revealed small arthritic spurring in the knees. I knew how important Cody's career was to him and to his countless fans. Wanting to not affect his ranking or performance, I wanted to avoid surgery if at all possible.

For his lower back pain, I tried epidural steroid injections for what seemed to be a lumbar disc degeneration. For the knees, I decided on a small steroid injection as well. On the day of the injection, Cody was a little nervous and was no longer sure he wanted to go ahead with the back injection. However, weighing the options between a needle prick and back pain, he decided to go through with them. I put him to sleep and performed the injections.

He awoke feeling no pain. Afterwards, he asked me why no one had ever suggested this to him before. I suggested that his doctors probably did not consider a nonsurgical option because it was so uncommon. Now, Cody is skating better than ever, doing his crazy stunts and keeping his fans happy.

Medial Collateral Ligament Syndrome

The medial collateral ligament is a flat, band-like ligament that runs from a portion of the femur known as the *medial condyle* to the long bone of the lower leg. The syndrome is usually the result of trauma, such as a fall with the leg in a rotated position, typical in ski accidents or in football clipping injuries. It is characterized by pain spreading all over the inside part of the knee, agitated by any rotation or flexing of the joint. The pain is constant and aching.

Diagnosis and Treatment

The medial collateral ligament feels tender when injured. Joint effusion and swelling may be present but can also suggest another condition, involving internal knee damage. An MRI and x-rays will help confirm a diagnosis.

As with arthritis, treatment includes nonsteroidal anti-inflammatory medications, physical therapy, and heat and cold application. Since activity involving the ligament may increase symptoms, it should be avoided. Injection of the medial collateral ligament with a local anesthetic combined with steroid medication can provide complete relief. Please refer to the website www.gotpaindocs.com, www.thegreatPainJack.com, or www.thegreatPainJack.org, for further information

> *Case Study:* *I treated Sharon, a very sickly workers' compensation injury patient. At twenty-nine she had already suffered a heart attack, a stroke, blockage and clotting of the large artery in her leg, and complications of diabetes, and had undergone several vascular bypass procedures. This young woman came to see me because of severe pain in her knee. Her difficult medical history precluded surgery and many medicinal therapies, especially since she also had allergies to a few of them.*
>
> *We tried a number of narcotics and nonnarcotic analgesics. All of them caused side effects such as drowsiness, constipation, and upset stomach. What ended up working for Sharon was a combination of simple injection therapy and a compounded concoction of medications specifically prescribed for her, including gabapentin, ketoprophen, ketamine, and lidocaine. These medications were made into a paste, which was then applied to her knees, relieving her painful knee condition.*

Suprapatella Bursitis

The suprapatella bursa travels beneath the knee. Injuries resulting from running on soft or uneven surfaces, or from crawling can cause suprapatella bursitis. The pain is located in the front of the knee and can travel up into the back of the thigh, preventing the sufferer from kneeling or walking down stairs.

Diagnosis and Treatment

Tenderness in the front of the knee is typical, as is swelling. The bursa may also feel hot to the touch. With overuse or trauma, the quadriceps muscle, i.e., the muscle primarily responsible for knee movement, and the suprapatellar bursa are subject to inflammation. Under strain, the tendons of the quadriceps muscle group unite to form a single very strong tendon, and anything that causes dysfunction of the quadriceps tendon can affect the suprapatella burse. Treatment of this condition involves anti-inflammatory medication, a knee brace to prevent further trauma, and, if the problem is not resolved, injection therapy.

Like the suprapatella bursa, the prepatella bursa, superficial infrapatella bursitis, and deep infrapatella bursitis are also vulnerable to injury from acute and repeated microtrauma. Sufferers of these conditions will complain of pain and swelling in the back of the knee. Kneeling and walking down stairs will cause immense pain, along with a sharp, catching sensation squat. Treatment should include anti-inflammatory medication and injection therapy. A knee brace should be prescribed as well.

Baker's Cyst

The Baker's cyst is a swelling in the knee, resulting from an accumulation of synovial fluid in the groove in the back of your knee. Often, a patient will not even realize he or she has a fluid-filled cyst behind the knee. When I call this to their attention, they are surprised. The swelling becomes more noticeable when a patient flexes the joint. The cyst may continue to grow or push fluid into the calf muscles. With frequent squatting, it can sometimes rupture spontaneously. The pain is characterized as aching and constant in nature, and can interfere with sleep.

Diagnosis and Treatment

X-rays are recommended for any patient that has swelling in the back of the knee. Nonsteroidal anti-inflammatory medication, an elastic band around the knee, and heat therapy are recommended as first-line treatments for the Baker's cyst. An injection with a local anesthetic and a steroid can also treat this condition. Surgery is extremely rare for removal of the Baker's cyst.

Pes Anserine Bursitis

The pes anserine bursa lies beneath the hamstring muscles. Patients with this syndrome will experience pain over the inside of the joint, aggravated by rotating the knee. Like other bursitis conditions of the knee, the pain is constant and aching in nature, resulting from overuse, misuse, or direct trauma.

Treatment

Conservative therapy consisting of analgesics, nonsteroidal anti-inflammatory medications, and knee bracing are reasonable first-line treatments. Injection therapy into the bursa is an excellent way to reduce a painful pes anserine bursitis.

Knee Pain Questionnaire–Answer these questions to map pain symptoms

*(Copy and fill out these worksheets and bring to your doctor. He/she may have his/her own, but answers to these questions provide a good overview of your pain condition and will help you remember and collect a **pain profile** in order to use your time with your doctor more effectively.)*

Where is your pain located?

When does your pain start and end?

When did you first begin to have pain, to the best of your recollection?

Where does your pain travel to?

Is it continuous throughout the day?

Has your pain ever improved?

Has it become chronic?

Are there two or more different types of pain syndromes that seem to occur simultaneously?

Does your pain wax and wane, or does it stay at the same intensity throughout the course of the day?

Does the pain occur all over?

Which pain bothers you the most?

Do the different pains that you have come from different areas and appear to be related to different conditions or movements of the face or body? Which pain would you like to get rid of the most?

Do you have a systemic disease diagnosed previously that may be contributing to your pain?

Do you believe your pain is caused by accident or injury?

Was this a work-related injury?

Could an old injury that did not heal be exacerbated by current daily activities?

Use the following scale to describe the severity of your pain for each type of pain you have,

with 1 being the least amount of pain and 10 being the highest level of pain you could ever imagine:.1 … 2 … 3 … 4 … 5 … 6 … 7 … 8 … 9 … 10.

What descriptors can you use for your pain: Burning? Aching? Shooting? Sharp? Throbbing? Cramping? Constant? Numbing? Lancinating? Stabbing? Transient? Excruciating? Tingling? On fire?

Does your pain get worse or better with sitting, bending, bending at the knees, lifting, walking, grasping, sweeping, standing, crawling, squatting, reaching overhead, eating, coughing, sneezing, physical activity, stress, driving, sexual intercourse, heat, ice, physical therapy, medications?

Have any of the following treatments provided relief of your pain condition: Surgery? Medications? Injection therapy? Chiropractic? Tens unit (electric stimulation)? Physical therapy? Traction? Heat therapy? Bed rest? Acupuncture? Psychotherapy?

Specific questions regarding knee pain to help you and your doctor make an accurate diagnosis

Does the knee pain seem to arise in the knee region primarily, or does it appear to come from another area that can be directed to the knee? _____

Is the knee pain fleeting, transient, or constant and throbbing? _____

Does the knee pain radiate down one or both legs? _____

Has the knee ever given out or buckled from under you? _____

If you have had knee surgery, do you still have pain coming from the same area? _____ A different area of the knee? _____

Is the knee pain associated with: Numbness? _____ Weakness? _____ Paralysis? _____ Increased or decreased sweating? _____ Skin discoloration? Skin rash anywhere on the face or body? _____ Tingling pins and needles on the neck or body? _____ Cold? _____ Muscle spasm? Tightness? _____ Trouble sleeping? _____ "Touch me not" pain? _____

What improves your knee pain? _____ What medications have you tried that failed? Have you had injections for your pain in the knee? _____ Have any of these modalities helped the knee pain: Sleep? _____ Rest? Ice? _____ Heat? _____ Pressure? _____ Exercise? _____ Any type of therapy? _____ Any kind of surgery? _____ Have you used light or laser therapy to try to treat your knee pain? _____ Do you use any rubs or topical agents to treat your knee pain? _____

What specific medications have you tried that failed? _____

What specific herbal or natural remedies have you tried? _____

Do you take supplements for your condition? _____

Is your knee pain accompanied with transient paralysis? _____ Do the muscles of your lower back go into spasm or become distorted at any time? _____ Do the knee or leg muscles appear to be weaker at any time? _____ Do the lower back muscles or the ability to hold the spine in position fail or tire easily? _____ _____

Body Map for Knee Pain Questionnaire

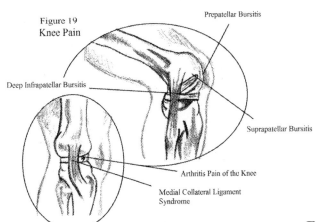

Figure 19
Knee Pain

Prepatellar Bursitis

Deep Infrapatellar Bursitis

Suprapatellar Bursitis

Arthritis Pain of the Knee

Medial Collateral Ligament Syndrome

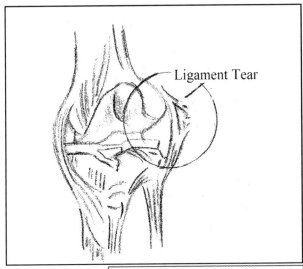

Figure 20
Knee Pain

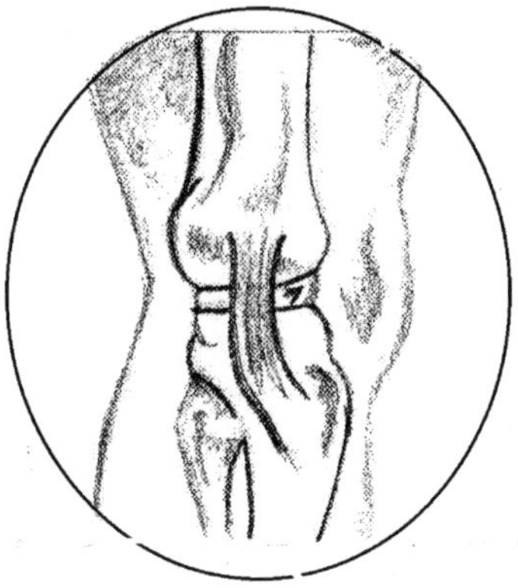

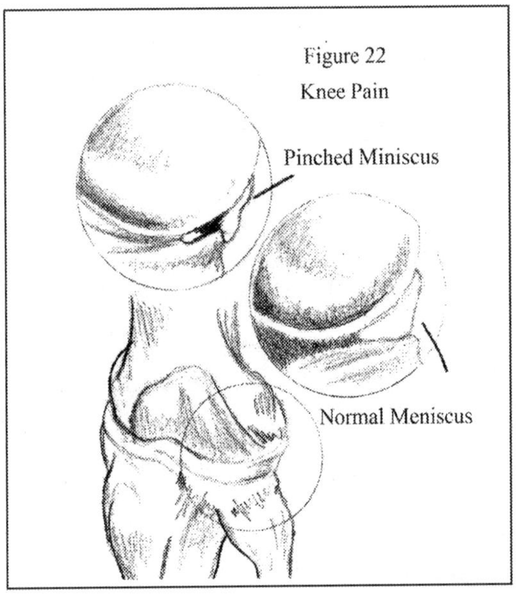

**Figure 21
Knee Pain**

Ligament Tear

Figure 22
Knee Pain

Pinched Miniscus

Normal Meniscus

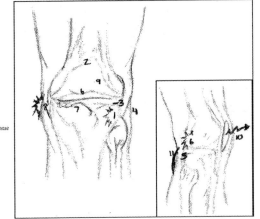

Figures 23 & 24
Knee Pain

1. Tibiofibular Pain Syndrome
2. Quadriceps Expansion Syndrome
3. Coronary Ligament Strain
4. Iliotibial Band Bursitis
5. Hamstring Tendinitis
6. Pes Anserine Bursitis
7. Arthritis of the Knee
8. Medial Collateral Ligament Syndrome
9. Suprapatellar Bursitis
10. Infrapatellar Bursitis
11. Baker's Cyst of the Knee

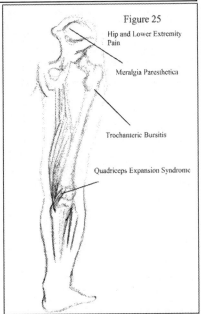

Figure 25

Hip and Lower Extremity Pain

Meralgia Paresthetica

Trochanteric Bursitis

Quadriceps Expansion Syndrome

Chapter 13:

So, You've Got Shoulder Pain?

Case Study: A woman (Bonny) came into the office as a new patient sobbing about how "no one cared about her" (condition) since she had fallen on hard times. She apparently had had neck surgery four months ago, which had not completely "cured" her condition. Additionally, she experienced some trauma (an assault and battery, I believe) where the long bone in her arm was shattered. The attempted surgical repair of the humerus (long bone in her upper arm) ended with a suboptimal result. She could barely move her arm, and the x-ray she brought along was actually embarrassing to look at. The surgical outcome performed years earlier was horrific. The bone was still shattered, with a long metal spike or rod run down the middle of the bone. The broken parts of the bone were still not connecting enough to allow for a surgical union. The operation was a failure. Bonny then underwent shoulder injection into the shoulder joint and subacromial space in anticipation of future shoulder surgery. She did eventually benefit from a cervical epidural, as neck pain was not completely treated by the previous neck surgery she had undergone. Some of the more common causes of shoulder pain include degenerative arthritis, acromioclavicular joint arthritis, subdeltoid or subacromial bursitis, bicipital tendinitis, rotator cuff tear, suprascapular nerve entrapment, and rotator cuff tendinitis. Please refer to the website www.gotpaindocs.com, www.thegreatPainJack.com, or www.thegreatPainJack.org, for further information.

Arthritis

Of the above, osteoarthritis, frequently a result of trauma, is the most common cause of shoulder pain. The pain from this condition is aggravated by activity. It is typically aching in nature and often is accompanied by popping or grinding when the shoulder is rotated. As the condition worsens, patients will experience a decrease in shoulder mobility.

Occasionally, causes of arthritis-induced shoulder pain may include collagen vascular diseases such as synovitis, Lyme's disease, and infection. If shoulder pain stems from infection, the sufferer will usually have a fever and feel weak.

Treatment

Arthritic shoulder pain should be treated with nonsteroidal anti-inflammatory drugs such as ibuprofen, cyclo-oxygenase inhibitors such as Celebrex, and physical therapy. For patients who do not respond to these measures, an injection of the shoulder with a local anesthetic and a steroid will produce significant reduction in symptoms for several months. A small number of these patients may feel an increase in pain after the injection before the relief sets in.

Bursitis and tendinitis are fairly common in people with arthritic shoulders. Specific localized injections into the bursa and tendons with an anesthetic and steroid will alleviate these two conditions. Heat and cold application can also help.

Acromioclavicular Joint Pain

The acromioclavicular (AC) joint, located above the shoulder, is extremely vulnerable to injuries, such as a fall directly onto the shoulder. Repeated strain from throwing injuries or raising the arms for a prolonged period of time, as when painting, can result in repetitive trauma to the AC joint. The joint may become inflamed, and, if the condition becomes chronic, arthritis may set in. Most patients are not able to sleep on the affected shoulder. They often complain of grinding and popping in the joint, especially when they wake up. The joint can swell and grow tender.

Diagnosis and Treatment

X-rays as well as an MRI are good tests to diagnose AC joint arthritis and ligament damage. An MRI will also differentiate if there is a shoulder abnormality, rotator cuff tear, AC joint abnormality, or biceps tendon injury. A physician should also perform a complete blood count, check the erythrocyte sedimentation rate, and do antinuclear antibody testing to test for rheumatoid arthritis and related inflammatory conditions.

Initial treatment associated with AC joint pain includes nonsteroidal anti-inflammatory drugs, cyclo-oxygenase two inhibitors, and physical therapy. Heat and cold application also helps. An injection of a local anesthetic and a steroid can supplement the above treatment.

Case Study: I often see patients with frozen shoulders from injuries sustained after falls and accidents. Injections into the shoulder joint as well as the acromioclavicular joint frequently cure this condition.

Randi, a forty-five-year-old woman with a known history of rheumatoid arthritis, scheduled for a total preoperative knee replacement, came in one day to see me and complained that she could not at all move her right arm. After careful examination, I did indeed discover degenerative osteoarthritis in her right shoulder, in addition to rheumatoid arthritis that affected most of the joints in her body. I suggested a simple steroid and anesthetic injection into the joint. She was morbidly afraid of needles but agreed.

Sure enough, after the injection she was able to move her arms and shoulders freely. This simple yet effective strategy can help countless sufferers with similar conditions.

Subdeltoid Bursitis

The subdeltoid bursa is also subject to injury from putting strain on the shoulders, working extensively with the arm above the body, repetitive motion associated with assembly line work, bowling, repetitive throwing injuries, and slips and falls.

Pain from subdeltoid bursitis is accentuated with movement of the arm away from the body. Typically people suffering from this condition will feel a catching sensation when moving the shoulder away from their bodies, especially in the morning. A sleep disorder is common this condition.

Diagnosis and Treatment

X-ray studies may reveal calcium in the subdeltoid bursa, which is generally associated with chronic inflammation. MRI studies may also diagnose conditions affecting the subdeltoid bursa such as tendinitis and disruption of the ligaments, and may diagnose associated rotator cuff tear. Nonsteroidal anti-inflammatory medication and physical therapy will reduce the symptoms. An injection into the bursa followed by gentle range of motion exercises, along with topical application of heat, may ease the patient's pain.

Biceps Tendinitis

The onset of biceps tendinitis is often sudden, resulting from overuse of the arm and shoulder joints. Injuries that can contribute to this condition include tennis serves or pulling motions such as starting lawnmowers. Pain from biceps tendinitis is constant and severe, and is located in the shoulder region. Many patients report sleep abnormalities.

Diagnosis and Treatment

Bursitis often accompanies biceps tendinitis, and occasionally with muscle atrophy a frozen shoulder may develop. As with other shoulder conditions, x-rays and an MRI of the affected limb helps make a diagnosis. Initial treatment should include nonsteroidal anti-inflammatory medication, physical therapy, and injections.

Case study: *A young athletic male, (Bobby Joe) came into the office complaining of shoulder* *and arm pain, abnormal temperature spikes, and feeling "sweaty" over the last two weeks. He had had a previous MRI that showed only mild biceps tendinitis. This was performed approximately four months previous. Apparently, he had undergone a procedure known as mobilization under anesthesia, in which the arm was "manipulated while he was under the influence of the anesthesia." He apparently did well after that, and about a month later he developed these unusual fevers and arm pain. A complete blood study was ordered, and a high white count was noted on his laboratory tests. This was fairly unusual, and the arm was very hot and tender. I became increasingly concerned and called his primary physician. His primary physician told me that he believed that the previous MRI did not reveal any specific findings, but he was concerned about the current clinical exam of the shoulder. I immediately told the primary care doctor that this gentleman needed an MRI arthrogram study to confirm what was going on in the shoulder. He reported to the hospital that evening and was admitted for over five days of treatment. He apparently became very sick and was treated with IV antibiotics for a necrotic bone mass inside the shoulder joint. Apparently this diagnosis had been missed previously, and now the young man, who had lost function of the arm, was struggling with surviving an episode of massive infection. A needle biopsy was performed, and a tissue sample was obtained for proper intravenous antibiotic treatment. He was provided medication and treatment in the hospital, but his insurance did not allow me to treat him at the hospital where he was admitted. Eventually the young man did have surgery to correct this problem of massive abscess cavity within the shoulder joint that originally presented with biceps tendinitis.*

Rotator Cuff Tear

Rotator cuff tears contribute to shoulder pain and dysfunction. Though this condition can be brought on by trauma to the shoulder, most often the real culprit is long-standing and untreated tendinitis.

The purpose of the rotator cuff is to rotate the arm and help provide the shoulder joint stability. The rotator cuff contains four muscle groups: *subscapularis, supraspinatus, infraspinatus,* and *teres minor* muscles. The supraspinatus and infraspinatus muscle tendons are particularly susceptible to tendinitis and inflammation. As the inflammation continues, calcium deposits may develop along the tendons. The shoulder will eventually lose range of motion, making everyday activities very difficult to perform.

Patients with a rotator cuff tear experience weakness after raising or rotating the arm. A partial rotator cuff tear implies the loss of smooth arm motion over the head, while a complete tear may lead to complete inability to raise the arm above the shoulder. Pain associated with rotator cuff tears is constant and severe. It is aggravated by raising the arm or rotating the shoulder.

Diagnosis and Treatment

X-rays as well as MRI studies should be performed if a rotator cuff tear is suspected. Since rotator cuff tears may occur after what appears to be just minor trauma, a diagnosis may have to be repeated. Failure to identify whether the tear is partial or complete will complicate the treatment. Usually this happens because an MRI study is not ordered at the outset. Rotator cuff tears rarely occur before the age of forty except in cases of severe acute trauma to the shoulder.

Anti-inflammatory medications along with an injection of anesthetic steroids are good initial treatments for people who have rotator cuff tears. Many times surgery will be indicated for a complete rotator cuff tear. However, the injection technique may work extremely well with partial rotator cuff tears or when surgery is not a viable option.

Case Study: A young carpenter, Hollis, came to my office one day to get a prescription for pain medication. A surfer (dude), with a long ponytail tucked up under his hat and a gentle demeanor had been on OxyContin for a large portion of his adult life for pain in his left shoulder. He had had surgery twice to correct a rotator cuff tear, a labral tear, and the degeneration of the shoulder cartilage. He had undergone a shoulder stabilization procedure as well, to keep the shoulder from migrating backwards into the shoulder cavity.

When I examined Hollis I grew astounded by how he had managed to compensate for what was essentially an immovable joint. Over time he had learned to use other muscles to compensate for those lost during previous surgeries. I examined the most recent MRIs and could not believe what I saw.

The tendons of the rotator cuff had completely given way and were now little more than frayed fibers. A condition known as the fatty infiltration of the muscle had developed. This was an ominous sign, as it usually implies that the affected muscle has become worthless and beyond surgical repair.

The supraspinatus tendon of his rotator cuff had been reduced to 5 cm, which meant there was nothing left to reattach it to the bone. I showed his MRI around the state, from San Diego to Sacramento, to see if I could get approval for a surgical remedy of his difficult condition. The response was unequivocal. No surgeon was willing to attempt to restorative surgery because of Hollis's prior failed operations.

Furthermore, the more time passed from the initial injury the more likely was further loss of function in Hollis's shoulder. Indeed, I soon found additional tears in the capsule of the shoulder joint, known as the labrum. The humeral head, also in the shoulder, became displaced. Time was of the essence.

I presented several options to him. On the one hand, a reverse shoulder implant could possibly restore some function, but all my consultants agreed that he would not be able to return to work as a carpenter. Tendon transfer surgery was also a possibility, as was composite grafting that could be sewn to the existing tendons, but with that amount of fatty infiltration of the now wasted muscle, neither option was ideal.

The jury is still out on this case. Hollis and I have decided on a series of occasional shoulder injections, with manipulation under anesthesia whenever his shoulder joint freezes up. Given his inability to take too much time off work to let any surgical procedure heal properly, this seems to be the best temporary solution. Unless he can find himself in a financial situation that will allow him to take the necessary time off work, Hollis will not be ready to fully heal.

Suprascapular Nerve Entrapment

Shoulder pain may arise from the entrapment of the suprascapular nerve, as seen in persons who frequently carry heavy backpacks. Patients typically complain of a severe, deep, aching pain that radiates from the top of the shoulder to the outer shoulder.

Diagnosis and Treatment

Electromyograms can help diagnose suprascapular nerve entrapment, as can x-rays and an MRI. Anti-inflammatory medications help to treat this condition. A local injection of the nerve with a steroid will minimize the symptoms. Occasionally surgical decompression of the suprascapular nerve may have to be performed if the aforementioned methods do not heal the patient. Please refer to the website www.gotpaindocs.com, www.thegreatPainJack.com, or www.thegreatPainJack.org for further information.

Supraspinatus and Infraspinatus Tendinitis

Both of these conditions occur in a younger group of patients following overuse or misuse of the shoulder joint. Examples of typical causes include throwing injuries, exercise equipment misuse, carrying heavy loads away from the body, or work-related assembly-line injuries. Chronic tendinitis of the supraspinatus and infraspinatus can occur in older patients. As with rotator cuff tear, as the disease progresses patients will generally lose shoulder function, making many of their daily activities very difficult.

Diagnosis and Treatment

As with other shoulder injuries, x-rays and an MRI are very helpful in making this diagnosis. Natural splinting may help minimize symptoms. Physical therapy, anti-inflammatory medications, and tendon injections will generally help treat the condition.

Case Study *A workers' compensation patient was referred to me for back pain that occurred as a result of an on-the-job injury. He was evaluated for lower back pain after he jumped* *from the cab on top of a truck and injured his shoulder in the process. Unfortunately he sustained a previous workers' comp injury in the form of a shoulder tear on another job.*

Because the previous claim was denied, I argued that the previous injury should be included in the current claim, as this was aggravated during the accident. The workers' compensation insurance company repeatedly denied the request, stating that it was the former carrier's responsibility.

The results of the first injury were shocking. Investigative medical work involved investigation into a head-on collision that occurred between two trucks on a freeway. The driver of the other truck was killed instantly. My patient sustained a shoulder injury in the crash. Unfortunately the shoulder injury, which was later determined to be a laberal tear, was never accepted as part of his medical condition. Therefore the insurance carrier repeatedly denied coverage for his shoulder.

As of the writing of this book, we still have not been able to get the necessary shoulder repair that would allow this patient to return to work. The two insurance companies keep arguing about whose responsibility it is to cover the injured shoulder from the head-on collision.

As far as the lower back is concerned, I was able to secure authorization to treat that in the form of epidural and facet injection. This caused modest improvement. It should be stated unequivocally that the patient will not recover from his overall condition unless the psychological aspects of the shoulder condition are treated.

The necessary treatment will likely involve psychological counseling as well as surgical repair. Often, in the medical compensation system the injured individual will be treated for only one body part and not many. This is not only illogical but can often lead to catastrophic settlements, because injured patients are denied care to thwart future and long-term chronic disabilities. If necessary treatments are provided relatively early, people will be less likely to injure themselves on the job in the future. An injured worker that has not received treatment for disability will not be able to provide solid work performance, particularly in the form of a trucker.

Injuries that are sustained on the job can be cumulative or immediate. In the case of this patient, his shoulder injury was immediate. Since previous treatment was denied and proper channels for treatment of the shoulder were not allowed, he went on to develop an additional condition in his lower back. Injuries of the lower back that were sustained in the second incident were allowed to be treated, but the vehement refusal by the insurance company stopped the treatment of the injured shoulder.

To date, this unfortunate individual is still in litigation involving the appropriate care and treatment of his condition. It is likely that surgery of the shoulder will be awarded; however, it is unclear that full recovery will ever occur. This is another example of how the psychological aspect of pain may affect a person's ability to heal. If the patient was granted proper treatment at an early phase, the psychological aspects of chronic pain would not necessarily be implicated.

Shoulder Pain Questionnaire–Answer these questions to map pain symptoms

*(Copy and fill out these worksheets and bring to your doctor. He/she may have his/her own, but answers to these questions provide a good overview of your pain condition and will help you develop a **pain profile** in order to use your time with your doctor more effectively.)*

Where is your shoulder pain located? _____

When does your shoulder pain start and end? _____

When did you first begin to have shoulder pain, to the best of your recollection?

Where does your shoulder pain travel to? _____

Is it continuous throughout the day? _____ Is the shoulder pain on both sides? _____

Has your shoulder pain ever improved? _____

Has it become chronic? _____

Are there two or more different types of pain syndromes that seem to occur simultaneously? _____

Does your shoulder pain wax and wane, or does it stay at the same intensity throughout the course of the day?

Does the shoulder pain occur all over? _____

Which shoulder pain bothers you the most? _____

Do the different shoulder pains that you have come from different areas and appear to be related to different conditions or movements of the face or body? _____

Which shoulder pain would you like to get rid of the most? _____

Do you have a systemic disease diagnosed previously that may be contributing to your shoulder pain? _____

Do you believe your shoulder pain is caused by accident or injury? Was this initially a work-related injury? _____

Could an old shoulder injury that did not heal be exacerbated by current daily activities? _____

Use the following scale to describe the severity of your pain for each type of pain you have, with 1 being the least amount of pain and 10 being the highest level of pain you could ever imagine: 1 … 2 … 3 … 4 … 5 … 6 … 7 … 8 … 9 … 10.

What descriptors can you use for your pain: Burning? Aching? Shooting? Sharp? Throbbing? Cramping? Constant? Numbing? Lancinating? Stabbing? Transient? Excruciating? Tingling? On fire?

Does your pain get worse or better with sitting, bending, lifting, walking, grasping, sweeping, standing, crawling, squatting, reaching overhead, eating, coughing, sneezing, physical activity, stress, driving, sexual intercourse, heat, ice, physical therapy, medications?

Have any of the following treatments provided relief of your pain condition: Surgery? Medications? Injection therapy? Chiropractic? Tens unit (electric stimulation)? Physical therapy? Traction? Heat therapy? Bed rest? Acupuncture? Psychotherapy?

Specific questions regarding shoulder pain to help you
and your doctor to make an accurate diagnosis

Does the pain seem to arise in the shoulder, or does it appear to come from another area (perhaps referred from the neck)? _____ What part of the shoulder causes the most pain: the front section, the top section, or the back section? _____

Is the shoulder pain fleeting, transient, or constant and throbbing? _____ _____

If you have had previous shoulder surgery, do you still have pain coming from the shoulder? _____ Have you had physical therapy after surgery? _____

Did this physical therapy help the condition? _____ Did it make it worse?

Is the shoulder pain associated with: Numbness? _____ Weakness? _____ Paralysis? _____ Increased or decreased sweating? _____ Skin discoloration? _____ Skin rash anywhere on the shoulder or body? _____ Tingling pins and needles on the shoulder or body? _____ Do you experience a cold sensation? _____ Muscle spasm or tightness? _____ Trouble sleeping? _____ "Touch me not" pain? _____

What improves your shoulder pain? _____ What medications have you tried that failed? _____ Have you had injections for your pain? _____ Is your pain improved by sleep? _____ By rest? _____ Ice? _____ Heat? _____ Pressure? _____ Exercise? _____ Any type of therapy? _____ Any kind of surgery? _____ Have you used light or laser therapy to try to treat your shoulder pain?

What specific medications are you using now? _____

What specific herbal or natural remedies have you tried? _____

Do you take supplements for your condition? _____

Is your shoulder pain accompanied by other symptoms? _____

How would you best describe these symptoms? _____

Is your shoulder pain accompanied with transient paralysis? _____ Do the muscles of your arm go into spasm or become distorted at any time? _____ _____

Does the affected shoulder appear to be weaker at any time? _____

Do you have a history of dropping items? _____ Inability to finish tasks such as sewing or crocheting? _____ hammering? _____ Difficulty in playing a game of tennis? _____ Difficulty in swinging a golf club? _____

Body Map for Shoulder Pain Questionnaire

Figure 26
Shoulder Pain

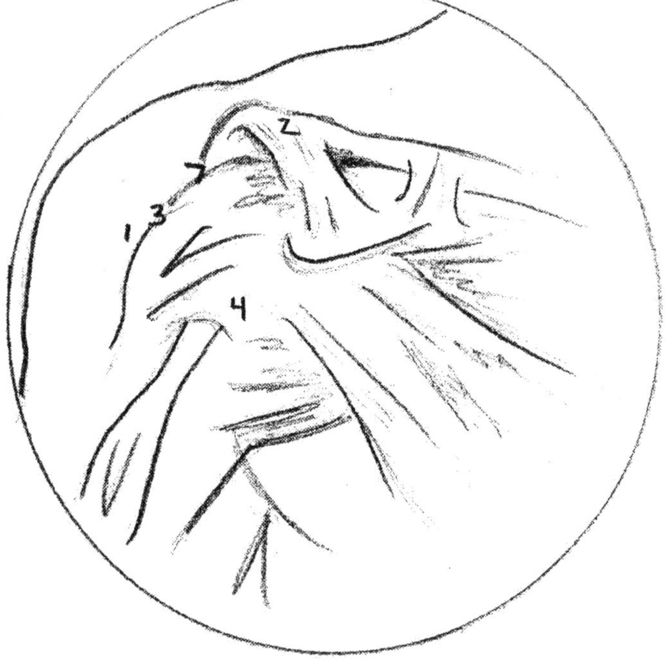

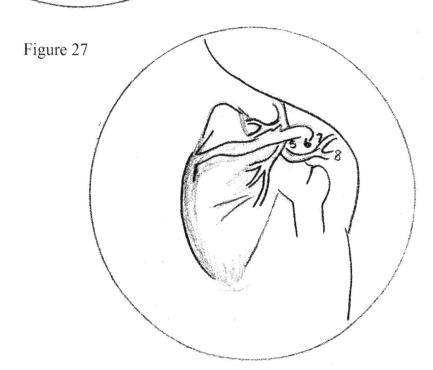

1. Arthritis of the Shoulder
2. Acromioclavicular Joint pain
3. Subdeltoid Bursitis
4. Bicipital Tendinitis
5. Rotator Cuff Tendinitis
6. Suprascapular Neuritis
7. Supraspinatus Tendinitis
8. Infraspinatus Tendinitis

Figure 27

Chapter 14

So, You've Got Fibromyalgia Pain?

A fibromyalgia diagnosis is much more common these days than, say, ten years ago, when it was considered a psychological condition existing in the patient's head. Today, it is considered a very real disease, not an imagined disorder. It derives its name from the Latin words *fibro*, meaning "fibrous tissue" such as tendons, *myo,* meaning "muscle," and *algia*, meaning "pain." Indeed, fibromyalgia affects soft tissues like muscles and causes widespread pain, fatigue, stiffness, and poor sleep, among many other complications.

Prevalence

The exact number of fibromyalgia cases is unknown, but it is estimated to exist in 5 percent of the world population. Though anyone can get it, women are approximately seven to ten times more likely to be diagnosed with fibromyalgia than men. The target age groups are usually between the mid-twenties and the mid-forties. According to Dr. Robert Bennett, a fibromyalgia researcher, approximately 35 percent of twenty-year-olds have fibromyalgia, while in a seventy-year-old population only about 12 percent have it.

Many people have fibromyalgia without knowing it. If you suspect you or a loved one has this condition, you should seek out a pain management specialist, rheumatologist, physiatrist, or a doctor of physical medicine and rehabilitation to make a diagnosis.

It is important to realize that many physicians do not want to treat fibromyalgia patients. There are several reasons for this bias. Some doctors simply do not understand or want to understand how to treat fibromyalgia patients. Similarly, and amazingly, considering the research done on the subject, many in the medical community believe that this disease entity is not real.

Symptoms

The main component of fibromyalgia is pain. It is typically located between the shoulder blades, the head, the neck, the lower back, and the hips. Though the pain affects primarily muscles, it also spreads to ligaments, tendons, or bursae, namely the air sacs between bones. These areas can become very tender and painful to the touch. More troublingly, the pain may move around to different sites on different days, a phenomenon known as "wandering pain." It can originate in one location, for example in a hip after a hard fall, and then gradually increase in severity and spread through the body so that the person doesn't even remember the inciting event. I often see this in young people after a car accident. Often, though the initial pain of this type of severe trauma is cured, pain may return and persist for years. Over half of the patients who have fibromyalgia attribute their symptoms to some type of trauma or severe stress.

When patients come to my office and I see on their intake sheet things like, "I feel like I've got run over by a truck," "I hurt all over," and "My pain moves all over my body," I consider a fibromyalgia diagnosis. Pain may be described as constant, aching, throbbing, and nagging. There may be generalized body aches all over, which may also be coupled with severe burning or stabbing pains in specific body parts. Other areas may have radiation patterns or lancinating qualities. The pain of fibromyalgia often interferes with everyday activities, affecting personal relationships and work.

Fibromyalgia may be exacerbated by weather changes. Cold, damp weather and cold drafts cause muscle pain to flare up. Cold water can have a similar effect. Heat and humidity can cause flare-ups.

Emotional stress negatively affects fibromyalgia patients as well. Women experience an increase in symptoms before their period begins, notably during the premenstrual syndrome (PMS). Pain symptoms can intensify during early menopause as well.

Fatigue is a common hallmark of the condition. It can vary in severity and can extremely limit a sufferer's activity. Some of my fibromyalgia patients call the office to tell me they know they have an appointment, but they simply cannot get out of bed. We know from research that fibromyalgia muscles have low energy storage and tire easily. Any activity can cause fatigue, which can also be unpredictable and affect the muscles suddenly. Recent research suggests that muscle fatigue may originate from the muscle spindle, which is part of a muscular motor unit in our skeletal muscles that allows us to move.

Extreme fatigue also has a mental component. *Neurasthenia*, the medical term describing extreme lack of energy and a feeling of mental exhaustion, makes it hard to focus on the task at hand. As a result, fibromyalgia can cause considerable difficulties with thinking, including forgetfulness, absentmindedness, confusion, and mental fatigue. Studies have shown that fibromyalgia patients exhibit a normal learning ability, but the processing of information may occur more slowly. For example, some patients will read the same thing over and over and not understand a word of what is written. Other patients can forget names, get lost while driving, or misplace items like keys around their house.

Poor sleep is also typical. Patients will often wake up tired, their sleep patterns characterized by frequent waking, especially in the early-morning hours. Others report trouble falling asleep, while they have no problem waking up. Headaches are also quite common. Tension, migraine, and combination headaches occur frequently in afflicted individuals.

Over a third of fibromyalgia patients feel pain in the jaw and temple areas. This pain may be related to temporomandibular joint dysfunction. A variety of symptoms such as headaches, facial numbness, spasm, flushing, swelling, and dizziness can result.

Patients with fibromyalgia have reported swallowing difficulties related to throat pain, swelling, and hoarseness. Symptoms of gastroesophageal reflux disease, in which stomach acid flowing back into the throat causes irritation, are common in fibromyalgia patients.

Neurologic symptoms such as numbness and tingling in the arms, legs, hands, and feet occur in fibromyalgia patients. Sensory abnormalities such as feelings of burning, itching, and swelling are common as well. Sometimes, a patient will experience insensitivity to temperatures. Attacks of vascular-related discoloration of the fingers or toes, known as Raynaud's phenomenon, are common in fibromyalgia patients, brought on by stress or cold temperatures. Sufferers also complain of vertigo, lightheadedness, dizziness, balance problems, and lack of coordination.

Fibromyalgic patients complain of dry eyes and are sensitive to smoke and dry air. The ocular muscles can have painful spasms, causing difficulty with focusing the eyes, tracking, or reading. Patients will change their prescription lenses frequently because of fibromyalgia-induced vision-related fluctuation.

Fibromyalgia can frequently cause chest pain. This is related to affected chest muscles rather than any coronary disease or angina. The diseased muscles become very tender and can mimic heart disease.

Joint pain and stiffness tend to exist with fibromyalgia. These symptoms are related to pain at the muscle and tendon insertions sites into the joint areas. Morning stiffness is a typical complaint, and many patients wake up in the morning feeling so stiff they can barely move.

Painful leg cramps, especially in the calves, are extremely commonplace. Generally occurring at night, they are relieved upon walking around. Sometimes a patient will suffer from *nocturnal myoclonus*, namely an involuntary jerking of the legs during sleep. These symptoms are exacerbated by a period of prolonged activity prior to sleep.

Allergic reactions to dust, pollen, colognes, smoke, medications, or foods occur more frequently in fibromyalgia patients. The significant increase in sinus headaches, nausea, itching, and nasal congestion is thought to be the result of an abnormally functioning allergic and immune system.

About half the fibromyalgia patients describe frequent bouts of constipation mixed with diarrhea. Irritable bladder and pelvic pain, as well as bladder infection with painful urination, are common.

As many as half the patients with fibromyalgia become clinically depressed. Depression can predate the diagnosis of fibromyalgia, and symptoms of low self-esteem, feelings of helplessness, and suicide attempts are not uncommon. Panic attacks and anxiety disorders may also be part of the fibromyalgic condition. Patients undergoing anxiety will usually experience a shortness of breath, racing heart, chest pain, and overt panic attacks.

Diagnosis

The presence of tender points is the main criteria to identify patients with fibromyalgia. According to a study by the American College of Rheumatology published in 1990, fibromyalgia is diagnosed when an individual has a history of widespread pain present for at least three months in at least eleven out of eighteen tender points in characteristic locations.

The pain is considered widespread if the following is true: the pain is in both sides of the body, and it is above and below the waist and along the spine. These are "signature areas" that distinguish individuals with fibromyalgia from those with chronic muscle pain and other causes. Please refer to the website www.gotpaindocs.com for further information.

The eighteen tender points are located in nine areas of the body, on both sides (hence eighteen). They include (1) the back of the scalp, (2) the low cervical muscles, (3) the trapezius muscle that extends from the neck to the shoulder, (4) the supraspinatus muscle located at the top of the shoulder blade, (5) a muscle right below the collarbone, (6) the lateral epicondyle located at the top of the forearm in the elbow, (7) the buttocks muscle, (8) the greater trochanter in the part of the thighbone with a protrusion right below the hip joint, and (9) the area above and inside the knee.

A positive tender point is one that is both tender *and* painful upon enough pressure to cause a thumbnail to blanch (equivalent to 4 kg of force). If the point is only tender, it is not a positive tender point. Mapping the tender points helps make the diagnosis and also aids in determining the type of treatment.

Conditions that mimic fibromyalgia include various types of arthritis, multiple sclerosis, and blood disorders. Laboratory tests, such as a complete blood count, sedimentation rate, thyroid function studies, and vitamin B12 levels can help differentiate some of these conditions from fibromyalgia.

Certain bodily chemicals will have abnormal levels in fibromyalgia patients. For example, serotonin, a hormone responsible for moods and concentration, is usually low in such patients. Substance P, a neurotransmitter responsible for transmitting and blocking of pain signals, is significantly higher in patients with fibromyalgia. Another chemical and brain hormone, Neuropeptide Y, is lower in patients with fibromyalgia, particularly under stressful conditions. This dysfunction will cause low blood pressure, anxiety attacks, and a rapid heart rate. Equally, fibromyalgia patients produce less cortisol, which helps us respond to and handle stress.

The excess of nerve growth may induce a hypersensitivity of the nerves, causing severe pain when the nerves grow or regenerate. This is common in patients who experience nerve trauma or spinal cord injury. However, in patients with fibromyalgia nerve growth may cause pain, even if there is no clear nerve injury.

I recall a very dear college friend who suffered bilateral nerve injuries in his arms and hands. He underwent a transplant of a donated kidney and pancreas due to childhood diabetes. After twelve hours of surgery, my friend woke up and could not feel or move his hands.

Most likely, during the surgery the bundle of nerves passing through the armpit (due to his positioning during the procedure), was injured. Since transplant surgery is extremely demanding, the focus of the surgeons is on the organs being transplanted rather than on the rest of the body.

It took over six months for my friend to regain partial function and sensation in his hands. During his nerve repair process, I'm certain that the nerve growth factor played a significant role in the burning and tingling pain he experienced during his rehabilitation.

A SPECT (single photon emission computerized tomography) scan is a study that evaluates brain function by measuring brain blood flow. Some researchers have identified abnormalities in parts of the brain in fibromyalgia patients involved in processing of pain.

Others have noted that there is an increase in the low-frequency brain waves in patients with fibromyalgia after experiencing trauma, which implies that the brain is functioning more slowly, and may explain symptoms of lack of focus, short-term memory less, and disorientation.

How It Works

Pain originates from nociceptors, which are specialized pain nerve endings. Tissue injury and damage to the muscles, soft tissues, and tendons activates the nociceptors. In cases of fibromyalgia, nociceptors continue to be activated, causing constant, severe, general pain. The disease causes nerves to become sensitized to the point of sending pain signals even in the absence of a stimulus. Now, the spinal cord becomes more sensitized to these pain signals and loses its ability to sort and filter them. Essentially, the nervous system is completely rewired by fibromyalgia. Different sensory signals, such as light, touch, temperature changes, pressure, and movement of the joints, become amplified and send pain signals to the brain.

To make matters worse, the brain's memory can store old pain. Fibromyalgia can cause previously injured areas to hurt more as it develops. Since fibromyalgia can amplify the pain pathways, it can awaken inactive old memories of previously injured body parts. The pain centers of the brain are mercilessly stoked with these amplified signals from the spinal cord. Brain waves change, serotonin levels decrease, and sleep is affected. Cognitive function is whipped to frenzy as the pain signals demand attention and energy in monitoring and filtering of their input. The patient is confused, disoriented, afraid, and depressed. And in pain.

Causes

A short list of fibromyalgia causes includes genetics, trauma, tissue diseases, infections, stress, chemical exposure, war, hormone disorders, and cervical spine stenosis. Genetically speaking, if a parent has fibromyalgia there is a 50 percent chance the child will get it too.

In predisposed individuals, physical trauma and tissue injury may lead to the development of fibromyalgia. Not surprisingly, in most physician practices, the most commonly reported trigger for fibromyalgia was trauma from car accidents, with work injuries being a close second.

Fibromyalgia may also be attributed to rheumatic and connective tissue diseases such as rheumatoid arthritis, systemic lupus, and autoimmune disorders such as thyroiditis, and systemic reaction to silicone breast implants.

Treatment

Treatment of fibromyalgia is based on three principles: (1) treating pain, (2) improving function, and (3) learning a successful program to self-manage the condition. Your treating specialist should help you achieve the highest quality of life with the least amount of pain possible. Learning about fibromyalgia through the Internet and perhaps joining a support group are two important ways of finding support once a diagnosis is provided.

Medications commonly prescribed to relieve symptoms of fibromyalgia include anti-inflammatory medication, analgesics, antidepressant medications, muscle relaxants, sleep medication, and antianxiety medication. Over-the-counter painkillers diminish the pain. Narcotic analgesics, such as Vicodin, Percocet, and OxyContin, can have negative side effects including respiratory depression, drowsiness, addiction, and impaired cognition. However, sometimes they are extremely necessary for patients with intractable pain.

Anti-inflammatory medication such as aspirin, nonsteroidal anti-inflammatory drugs such as ibuprofen, and steroid medications such as prednisone may be helpful in reducing pain that flares up after increased physical activity and muscle strain. As a side effect, these drugs can cause gastrointestinal bleeding.

Antidepressants and selective serotonin reuptake inhibitors such as Prozac or Zoloft can treat mood disturbances and sleep problems. The selective reuptake inhibitors also treat depression by blocking the breakdown of serotonin. Their negative side effects may include sexual dysfunction, sluggishness, and weight gain.

Muscle relaxants can alleviate muscle pain associated with fibromyalgia. Antispastic agents such as Zanaflex and Baclofen have been shown to reduce muscle back spasms and pain.

Sleep medication, while habit-forming and a potential cause of rebound insomnia, can improve deep sleep when taken appropriately. Benzodiazepines such as Xanax are commonly used for sedation and sleep. Negative side effects include memory impairment and depression. One of these drugs, Klonopin, can be particularly useful in treating the restless leg syndrome condition.

A series of trigger point injections can be administered to reduce pain and spasms—a relief that can last for weeks. These are generally benign and are performed with very small needles. Also, BOTOX injections can be beneficial in people who are resistant to trigger point injections. Other types of therapeutic injections that may be particularly helpful, particularly when other conditions coexist, include epidural steroid injections, selective nerve root block injections, joint injections, tendon injections, and prolotherapy. Prolotherapy is a technique where stimulatory substances are injected into injured tissue to promote a specific response.

Fibromyalgia patients should avoid nicotine, caffeine, alcohol, and artificial sweeteners. Generally, a fibromyalgic patient's diet should include high-protein and low-carbohydrate foods. Nutritional supplements such as magnesium, malic acid, vitamins B6, B1, and C, manganese, and colostrum can help treat fibromyalgia.

B12 injections promote generalized health, energy, and improvement of immune functions. Since B12 is not absorbed well when taken orally, it should be administered via injection.

Glucosamine and chondroitin, as well as methyl sulfonyl methane, are natural products that aid in repair and regeneration of cartilage and ligaments. They can reduce inflammation as well as improve hormone and protein function.

Natural serotonin producing supplements such as St. John's wort can help the body produce serotonin. Natural sleep modifiers such as valerian root and melatonin can be used as natural sleep aids and stress relievers.

Antioxidant therapy with immune boosters and vitamin C, zinc, echinacea, cinnamon, garlic, and goldenseal can help boost immune function. Many of these products can be found in your local grocery store, but please make sure you read the label for ingredients when prescribed antioxidant therapy by your doctor. Antioxidants in general are used to help target free radical formation, support cellular functions, and improve the immune function of natural killer cells. Other common antioxidants include vitamins A and E, grape seed extract, resveratrol (found in red wines), and lipoic acid. Licorice root and ginseng can also improve adrenal gland function and support stress responses by replenishing the stress hormones.

General fibromyalgia questionnaire–Answer these questions to map pain symptoms

*(Copy and fill out these worksheets and bring to your doctor. He/she may have his/her own, but answers to these questions provide a good overview of your pain condition and will help you remember and develop a **pain profile** in order to use your time with your doctor more effectively.)*

Where is your fibromyalgia pain located? _____

When does your fibromyalgia pain start and end? _____

When did you first begin to have pain, to the best of your recollection? _____ _____

Where does your fibromyalgia pain travel to? _____

Is it continuous throughout the day? _____

Has your fibromyalgia pain ever improved? _____

Has it become chronic? _____

Are there two or more different types of pain syndromes that seem to occur simultaneously? _____

Does your fibromyalgia pain wax and wane, or does it stay at the same intensity throughout the course of the day? _____

Does the pain occur all over? _____

Which fibromyalgia pain bothers you the most? _____

Do the different fibromyalgia pains that you have come from different areas and appear to be related to different conditions or movements of the face or body? _____

Which fibromyalgia pain would you like to get rid of the most? _____

Do you have a systemic disease diagnosed previously that may be contributing to your pain? _____

Do you believe your fibromyalgia pain is caused by accident or injury? Was this initially a work-related injury? _____

Could an old injury that did not heal be exacerbated by current daily activities?

Use the following scale to describe the severity of your pain for each type of pain you have, with 1 being the least amount of pain and 10 being the highest level of pain you could ever imagine: 1 … 2 … 3 … 4 … 5 … 6 … 7 … 8 … 9 … 10.

What descriptors can you use for your pain: Burning? Aching? Shooting? Sharp? Throbbing? Cramping? Constant? Numbing? Lancinating? Stabbing? Transient? Excruciating? Tingling? On fire?

Does your pain get worse or better with sitting, bending, lifting, walking, grasping, sweeping, standing, crawling, squatting, reaching overhead, eating, coughing, sneezing, physical activity, stress, driving, sexual intercourse, heat, ice, physical therapy, medications?

Have any of the following treatments provided relief of your pain condition: Surgery? Medications? Injection therapy? Chiropractic? Tens unit (electric stimulation)? Physical therapy? Traction? Heat therapy? Bed rest? Acupuncture? Psychotherapy?

Specific questions regarding fibromyalgia pain to help you and your doctor to make an accurate diagnosis

Does the fibromyalgia pain seem to arise in the neck and upper back or does it appear to come from another area (perhaps referred from the neck or head)? _____ What part of the body causes the most pain? _____

Is the fibromyalgia pain fleeting, transient, or constant and throbbing? _____ _____

If you have had previous surgery, do you still have pain coming from the body part? _____ _____ Have you had physical therapy after surgery? _____

Did this physical therapy help the condition? _____ Did it make it worse? _____

Is the fibromyalgia pain associated with: Numbness? _____ Weakness? _____ Paralysis? _____ Increased or decreased sweating? _____ Skin discoloration? _____ Skin rash anywhere on the trunk or body? _____ Tingling pins and needles on the shoulder or body? _____ Do you experience a cold sensation? _____ Muscle spasm or tightness? _____ Trouble sleeping? _____ "Touch me not" pain? _____

What improves your fibromyalgia pain? _____ What medications have you tried that failed? _____ Have you had injections for your pain? _____ Is your pain improved by sleep? _____ By rest? _____ Ice? _____ Heat? _____ Pressure? _____ Exercise? _____ Any type of therapy? _____ Any kind of surgery? _____ Have you used light or laser therapy to try to treat your fibromyalgia pain? _____

What specific medications are you using now? _____

What specific herbal or natural remedies have you tried? _____

Do you take supplements for your condition? _____

Is your fibromyalgia pain accompanied by other symptoms? _____

How would you best describe these symptoms? _____

Is your fibromyalgia pain accompanied with transient paralysis? _____

Do the muscles of your arm go into spasm or become distorted at any time? _____ _____

Does the affected body part appear to be weaker at any time? _____

Do you have a history of dropping items? _____ Inability to finish tasks such as sewing or crocheting? _____ hammering? _____ Difficulty in playing a game of tennis? _____ Difficulty in swinging a golf club? _____

Body Map for Fibromylagia Questionnaire

Figure 26
Shoulder Pain

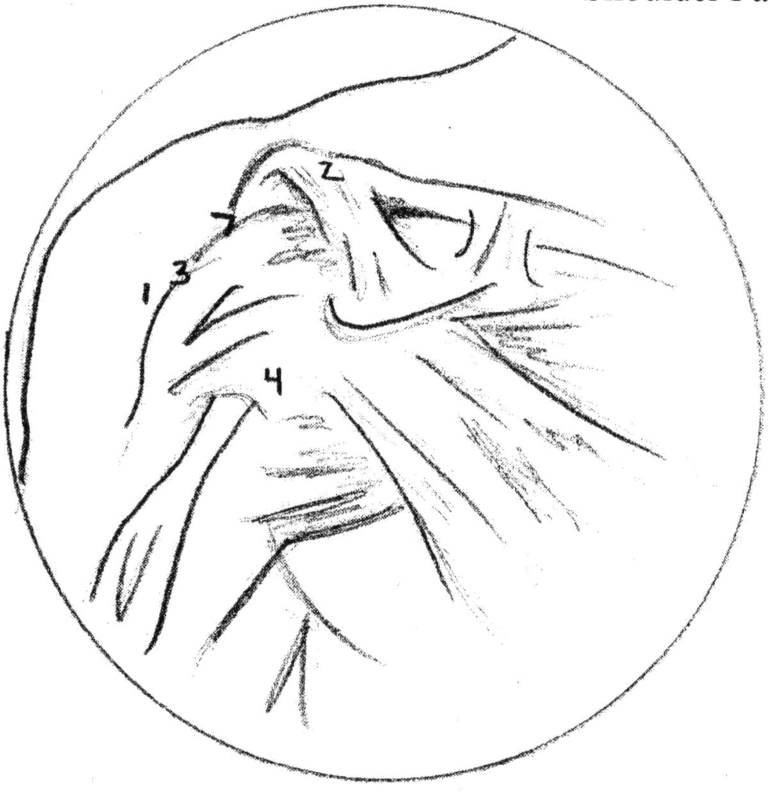

1. Arthritis of the Shoulder
2. Acromioclavicular Joint pain
3. Subdeltoid Bursitis
4. Bicipital Tendinitis
5. Rotator Cuff Tendinitis
6. Suprascapular Neuritis
7. Supraspinatus Tendinitis
8. Infraspinatus Tendinitis

Chapter 15:

The Psychology of Pain

*P*sychological Aspects of Healing: *I was covering a hospital shift one day, and I was told that a thirty-seven-year-old woman, who had given birth to a healthy boy four months earlier, was diagnosed with colon cancer. It was not clear if it was metastatic at the time, but arrangements for special catheter insertion to administer chemotherapy were made during her upcoming surgery.*

All in all, a seven-hour operation prevailed in which a large segment of her colon was removed. Lymph node dissections were also carried out, as well as placement of an IV catheter, and a biopsy of a rectal mass was made. It was unclear as to why this type of cancer would affect this woman at such a young age.

I remember that prior to the surgery she asked me to ask the anesthesiologist and other support members of her care, including the surgeons, to read certain affirmations during the procedure. I agreed to this request and read the affirmations while she was under general anesthesia. I'm not sure there were any direct effects of the reading, but I am quite certain that her belief in that her caregivers wanted her recovery and performed her request indeed contributed to helping her along the healing process. I also offered to place an epidural catheter for pain relief from the seven-hour operation. She was delighted that she woke up from the operation essentially pain free and that in a reasonable amount of time she was able to resume breast-feeding her baby. (Providing epidural medication in the form of narcotics would mean that less narcotics would have to be in her system and therefore would be less likely to cross over into the breast milk and affect her baby.)

She thanked me for this. She would have probably suffered grave psychological manifestations of pain, but due to her overwhelming support system in the form of a very spiritual and supportive family I feel that she was afforded the best opportunity to make a recovery that could be provided. In this type of nurturing and healing environment it is very clear that psychological aspects of her pain and ultimately her condition, which would require chemotherapy, could be controlled well.

It is this attitude that rendered her immune system with the best possible defenses to fight off any existing cancer cells that may not have been removed during the surgery. If the immune system is affected in a positive way it is likely that powerful immune modulators will suppress any additional type of cancer cell formation in her body.

One of the main reasons why we feel pain is to help us avoid danger, real or perceived. Also, pain results in the modification of behavior that will prevent future injury, without which carrying of the species would not be possible. Pain essentially plays a survival mechanism role in that it can resurface as a memory, either learned firsthand or passed on through ancestors or parents that can be protective and/or preventative against future injury.

Now taking this a step further, unfounded fear and the pain associated with it can lead to anxiety and generalized anxiety disorders, which also can be construed as providing the basis for neuroses. Psychological pain can then have a deep and lasting impact on imprinting. Imprinting is an experience that is usually associated with high emotion. And this often creates lasting memories deep within the limbic system where the emotional centers that control behavior are located.

The memory of pain and the reason for the essence of pain then mixes with thought processes that are processed in the forebrain, in the cognitive part, and the experience of pain is then modulated. Now, cognitive thoughts can accentuate or diminish those memories of pain. For example, in the survival mode, if a child is nearly hit by a bus as it approaches a bus stop, a delay in the reaction of a parent will create an imprinting event on that child's psyche.

In essence, the painful experience associated with this near miss episode may be interpreted later in life in another way. Life experiences may then modify the essential pain experience. That is not to say that the individual will need psychotherapy to unwind the pain emotional substructure of the event, but depending on the intensity of the emotion of the imprinting event, the psychological aspect of pain will be affected.

Depression: *A woman came to me complaining of headaches and neck pain. Her family brought her in because she was falling asleep due to overuse of medications taken during the day. Soon we identified the cause of her intractable pain. She was found to have degenerative spine disease and underwent a detox program ordered by me. She successfully returned to a normal level of medications that controlled her pain. However, she was still unable to improve her symptoms with injection therapy alone.*

She underwent neurosurgical treatment for her condition. She did well for approximately one year after the surgery and no longer needed my services for detoxification. The patient was released to her primary care physician, and she continued to apparently do well. However, in a tragic twist of fate, perhaps due to a lack of medication, and despite all the appearances of being healed, she drove her car into a tree and killed herself.

This is an example of how, despite every effort to treat the patient appropriately, the treatment can give rise to depression, which needs to be treated separately and distinctly. If the patient's depression had been treated she would not have seen such a tragic end. This underscores the need for treatment of depression that may accompany chronic pain and for a multimodal approach with disciplined specialists in different fields to treat the various segments of pain.

In dealing with pain in a clinical setting, often the average chronic pain management clinic will overlook these essential points in treatment and therapy. In our clinic we deliberately seek a history of the overall pain experience. The history can delve into childhood misfortune, such as deep emotional traumatic events. The experience of pain associated with a childhood event may be repressed, and it may be in effect to elicit this history.

Some disease states are associated with traumatic events, such as a car accident, for example. Conditions such as fibromyalgia are known to have high association with car accidents and/or with child abuse or trauma.

A painful experience suffered early on in life can lead to a modulation of protein structure and the maturation of the immune system. The immune system is the main policing system in our bodies. Pain and the chronic pain experiences, and the high cortisol stress hormone, can negatively affect the ability of immune cells to rid the body of cancer cells and bacteria, and can affect antibacterial and antiviral action. The immune system is so highly affected by a person's psychological state that numerous studies have demonstrated the beneficial effect from positive reenforcement of thinking in battling various disease entities.

One example where a development of a disease condition may be affected by a psychological painful experience would be the onset of juvenile diabetes, which typically occurs between ages seven and thirteen. There is the emotional state associated with an adverse effect on the immune system that may render the eyelet of Langerhands cells incompetent. That is to say, the cells of the pancreas that create insulin are adversely affected by a viral entity that would normally be attenuated and rendered harmless by a healthy immune system. If a negative experience is associated with immune suppression at or about the time the virus may attack the cells of the pancreas, juvenile diabetes may result. Occasionally, in interviewing juvenile onset diabetics, a memory of a very torrid or traumatic event can be associated with the onset of diabetes.

In treating a somatic pain syndrome or disease entity, it is therefore important to establish a bond with the mental substrate of an individual in identifying a psychological perception of pain. If the individual that is afflicted is of the understanding that a qualified practitioner is indeed trying to heal the overall aspect of the pain experience, then therapy is more likely to be successful. If, on the other hand, the individual does not believe the pain practitioner or physician has a vested interest in hearing the psychological aspect of pain, and shows indifference to the patient's dilemma, it is unlikely that a resolution to the pain experience will occur.

For this reason, multidisciplinary pain syndromes have created a model where psychologists, psychiatrists, and counselors alike are involved in the management of the psychological pain experience. Without healing of the mind, there is no healing of the body. Nothing can be more appropriately said when it comes to true healing. True healing will only occur when an individual submits his or her true pain experience to a pain practitioner who can truly understand the sequence of events that led to a chronic pain condition.

Battered Woman Syndrome: *Recently I was alerted to a car accident that was well-publicized in the local news. It involved a collision between a bus and an SUV. The SUV was driven by an underage, drunk driver. He and all his passengers were killed.*

I had the sheer horror of hearing the story recounted firsthand to me by one of the victims that was inside the bus, which was propelled end-over-end at three thirty. on a July morning.

The SUV rolled over and was blocking the freeway. The bus, driving on a freeway in the central valley in California, swerved at the last minute to try to avoid contact with the SUV. However, it was not able to maintain control and twisted and turned violently in the air. Then, after coming to a stop, it was hit by another SUV that was coming from the rear, which caused a third impact. Finally the bus became lodged in an embankment along the freeway.

A twenty-nine-year-old woman was traveling with her eight-year-old son on the bus that day. She described to me, with sheer horror, the bracing and protective maneuvers she made to try to protect her son from harm. She sustained injuries to her neck, head, and lower back, and had leg and facial fractures, including her nose.

As of the writing of this book she is still under treatment and will require psychological counseling. Psychological counseling is the likely aspect of her care that will do the most good for her at this time. However, it was unfortunately denied by her regular health insurance as well as by the litigation that was associated with this bus accident.

In a surprising twist, I learned that this young woman, Mrs. S——, was a victim of domestic abuse and was actually fleeing to a safe house in another city. In an effort to flee that relationship she sought refuge in another city and ended up on the bus that weekend with her son. She believed she was on her way to safety and had no idea what horrible future was awaiting her.

She described vividly how she was able to cover her son during the violent twisting and torquing in the bus. She described how she was helped by other passengers to climb out the bus window after it rolled on its side in the ravine next to the freeway. Bruised, badly injured, and shaken, she was taken to the local hospital. There, the hospital diagnosed no specific fractures except a nasal fracture and a urinary tract infection. The doctors did not offer any antibiotics for the urinary tract infection. They recommended she see her local doctor as soon as possible.

Unfortunately this is the fate of many accident victims after attempting to get treatment at local emergency rooms. Emergency rooms are typically overwhelmed, and, unless there's catastrophic injury such as lung/bone fractures, lung injuries, or abdominal organ injuries, hospitals try to limit less severe types of admissions.

Fortunately, Mrs. S—— did not have to return to the house she fled. Alternative housing arrangements were made for her and her son. What struck me as very remarkable was that although this woman was very severely injured in the accident, it appeared that she did not display an inordinate amount of suffering and pain. This could be because of psychological intervention that had occurred early. It also might have been because she could be suffering from battered woman syndrome.

This syndrome occurs when an abused woman internalizes feelings of punishment and abuse. Thus the victim suffers doubly. On the one side, she suffers from the domestic abuse, and, on the other side, the physical signs and manifestations of abuse are hidden because of mixed feelings of love, forgiveness and punishment that race through the afflicted woman's mind.

It isn't clear if battered woman syndrome plays a significant role in the scale-down of this individual's physical injuries sustained in the bus crash. It is clear, however, that she will need surgery to at least repair her fractured nose, which is significantly displaced and causes disfigurement of her facial features.

I've often been told by patients that I'm the only doctor who understands their situation. I say this not to be boastful, but it appears that sharing with submission of the pain experience is indeed part of the natural healing therapy. It can be associated with a multimodal approach. Occasionally, in intense therapy, a patient will reveal very personal secrets and relinquish this information as if he or she had been waiting years to tell someone, but no one was around to listen. I suggest that, with the breakdown of the family unit and with the electronic communication of our current society, conversation and the emotional release that is associated with talking about the pain experience have been thrown by the wayside. This experience, known as catharsis, is the total release of emotions and the purging that occurs when the pain experience is gotten off of one's shoulder.

The reason for catharsis may have its roots in the fact that there is no one there typically to listen to a patient's pain condition. Oftentimes these pain conditions run on for years with a multitude of symptoms, trial diagnoses, and varied symptom complexes. When, finally, a practitioner that understands pain is able to relate to the pain experience and understand, diagnose, and treat the condition, the patient's emotional release is tremendous.

There are individuals for whom catharsis may not be possible in treatment. There is a basis for this phenomenon. Occasionally patients will make up symptoms to achieve a secondary goal or are not able to articulate their pain experience. I've seen this in individuals who have brain damage, either through trauma, the usage of recreational drugs, or other injuries.

The nonverbal chronic pain patient has a difficult time because most of his or her pain experience is internalized. The internalization of the pain experience does not lead to complete healing. It is also for this reason I firmly believe that group therapy sessions can be beneficial to chronic pain sufferers. Group therapy serves as a support network for like chronic pain sufferers, a support group for people who, for example, experience posttraumatic stress disorders or fibromyalgia. Support group therapy can also prevent relapses. The members help each other stop misusing their medications, for example. They also make the chronic pain sufferers feel less alone in their suffering. Humans are social beings, and they seek others for acceptance and comfort. The group environment may, as a result, prevent relapses. Please see www.gotpaindocs.com, www.thegreatPainJack.com, or www.thegreatPainJack.org for additional information.

Chronic pain sufferers will come to the clinic with no specific diagnosis and no health insurance. The sense of abandonment they experience can create huge difficulty in providing diagnosis and treatment. We do not turn away patients for not having insurance, but a lot of other clinics do, which results in a large group of patients who need mental and medical health care, just like everyone else. We provide our patients with psychological and spiritual counseling, detoxification programs, and reading materials to enable them to make their own decisions about managing their pain condition.

Patients who have been through other pain clinics often find these services overwhelming, in that they are offered more than they expect. A twenty-four-year-old entering a clinic with PTSD from service in Afghanistan and with combat injuries, who seeks an OxyContin prescription, doesn't necessarily need this sort of therapy. In situations such as this I will recommend a free counseling session at the clinic. This may involve a specialist, like an interventionalist, or a person of a religious background, such as a priest or a rabbi.

As a result of these interventions, I have been thanked countless times by individuals who were used to being dismissed with a drug prescription. It is this element of surprise that can often build strong bonds between the patient and the doctor. For individuals who, due to their pain, lost meaning in their life, the thought of speaking to one of our specialists is completely mind-blowing. Patients who have ulterior motives and who search for drug prescriptions may change their perspective on their needs.

Psychological aspects of pain are as important as the somatic and physical aspects. The provider with true wisdom seeks to promote healing in all of these areas.

Pain and Psychology: *An attractive young woman, Ms. F——, came to see me regarding something very disturbing. She said she was hurting in different parts of her body, including her chest and back. I began asking some standard questions about the quality, and everything proceeded fairly normally. That is until I asked her about possible causes of her pain.*

Ms. F—— then began talking about her ex-husband.

She spoke calmly, with a foreign accent and a profound attention to detail. She told me that her husband subjected her to "sinister torture methods," applying "shock-like devices" to various portions of her body. She went on to say that her ex-husband learned the techniques while in an undisclosed Middle Eastern country, where he worked with the FBI and CIA. He violently abused her like this, beating and torturing her, over the course of a few years. When I asked her where it hurt the most, she pointed to her chest, then her heart.

After she finished her story, I remember looking at this beautiful young woman, who did not resemble at all the torture victim she described, and being in shock. All of what she told me took time to sink in.

I began examining her case further. I asked her about her medical history. She told me that she had been hospitalized for an extended period of time, during which she was extensively tested for various types of medical conditions. All the results pointed to a relatively benign diagnosis, even though F—— was convinced her ex-husband had caused permanent nerve damage.

I asked if she had access to these studies, wanting to verify her story. She told me she did not. I asked where the ex-husband was and if she felt safe. F—— said she had moved back with her mother, and he was not around. Then she paused. She looked at me. She admitted that she often felt like he was stalking her and that her house was possibly "bugged."

I looked at her prescription medications and learned that she had been to a psychiatrist, who treated her for delusional behavior. Indeed, F—— was incredibly convincing. It became clear to me, however, that her ability to persuade others was so successful because she herself clearly believed that the events she described had taken place.

With this new piece of information, I was no longer sure how much of what she was telling me was true and how much was fabricated. I called in my own pain psychologist to help. Mistakenly I believed that a female pain psychologist would be more effective at talking to F——, but I was wrong; she preferred males.

I was stuck, unable to substantiate her story. This was not the first time someone had told me that she has been implanted with devices by the FBI or the CIA or some other government entity. Thus, over time, I learned not to interrupt or criticize but to listen. And so I listened intently, and compassionately, to her wild stories, which she told in great detail, offering me her mind's understanding of her sordid past.

I tried not to dwell on her past, focusing rather on how to go about healing her. However, if I was going to attempt any time of therapy to improve her state of mind, it was important to establish a bond with her.

As the months passed, I put her on medication that clearly helped alleviate her pain. But my focus was always on establishing a safe forum for her to feel comfortable to purge her past traumatic memories. I knew this would take time.

I began exploring different healing therapies, including low-intensity laser therapy, light therapy, an ultrasound, and massage therapy. I could see a change in Ms. F——. She began to look forward to our monthly sessions and became more engaged in my recovery plan for her. I prescribed her walks and a specific exercise program. I also firmly believed that her mental condition warranted a delicate balance of medication in the form of analgesics, muscle relaxants, tranquilizers, and antipsychotics.

Soon she grew more comfortable with the treatment, and I started weaning her off the medications, leaving only a small safety net in case she had a setback. Essentially, I continued to have her seek emotional and psychological counseling at our clinic as I reduced her dosage. I wanted Ms. F—— to believe that the treatment designed for her had a chance of working. If she doubted it, the treatment would be doomed to fail.

Anecdotal reports in medical literature are full of failed medical therapies for one reason or another. What most physicians tend to forget is how crucial a patient's embrace of a treatment plan is to its success. This shouldn't be mistaken with the placebo effect; the patient simply gives the treatment a chance, following its prescriptions to a T.

Ms. F—— told me she did not trust any of the previous treatments doctors prescribed for her. I asked her what type of therapy she thought could treat her condition. She told me she believed over-the-counter, medicated patches could help her, as well as a return to her native Mexico.

I had a profound realization. I suddenly understood that surgery, epidural steroid injections, massage, or chiropractic would not really benefit her because she did not believe in their potential for success. Perhaps she was right. Much to the chagrin of other doctors involved in her care, I recommended that we prescribe the treatment she believed would make her better.

Another woman, Maria, was injured in a work-related incident and had terrible cervical spine stenosis. She needed neck surgery but refused treatment, not believing that the surgery would help her. I asked her what she believed would help her. She believed that over-the-counter patches for pain relief would cure her.

So I recommended the over-the-counter patches and a return to Mexico for an extended sojourn. Maria was elated when I approved this treatment plan. She returned to her native land, and I later heard she was doing well, happy and healthy. I recommended nonsurgery for this individual because she did not believe the surgery would help her. Who was I, her treating doctor, to demand she undergo surgery if she did not believe it would help?

The Placebo Effect

The placebo effect plays a large role in pain management. It has been defined as a physiologic effect caused by a placebo, with its roots largely in the psychology of the patient. It involves multiple issues. For one, a doctor who is trusted by the patient and who fosters a good bond with him or her is extremely important. The placebo effect is essentially a cure of the mind, which is a subjective extension of the pain experience. This suggests that belief itself is powerful medicine, even if the treatment itself is a sham.

In the past, placebos have helped alleviate pain, depression, anxiety, Parkinson's disease, inflammatory illnesses, and even cancer in some reported instances. The biology and chemistry of the placebo effect suggest that the responses to placebos stem from the brain. The effect comes not only from the belief in the drug procedure's ability to treat the condition but also comes from the subconscious associations between recovery and the existential experience of being treated. This brings us back to the compassionate physician who adds the extra ounce of medicine to his diagnostic and therapeutic regimen by holding a hand, sporting a smile, or lending a personal touch to the treatment.

In my clinic we have expanded on this idea to include such experimental options as a thoughtful prayer, encouragement e-mails, booster tweets, or supplementation of patient visits with health-care and non-health-care practitioners. It is my fundamental belief that if patients believe they are treated with dignity and utmost attention, their road to recovery and their ability to cope with pain drastically improves.

Daily tweets and electronic messages such as text and e-mail can boost this belief system. It can be demonstrated that when patients know their doctor is 100 percent behind their treatment and cure, recovery can proceed at a much faster rate. Furthermore, the personal touch of knowing that a pain management provider, psychologist, or other health professional is 100 percent behind the treatment will allow for subliminal conditioning, which can control bodily processes such as immune response and the release of healing hormones. That is not to say these things will cure the disease, but they do not have a negative impact.

The power of positive influence and a strong provider, leader, and coach is necessary in the treatment of patients with chronic pain syndromes. These patients often have attendant psychological conditions, such as depression, anxiety, and so on. The doctor can alleviate these through his leadership in the treatment process.

For many patients, the comorbidity of dealing with cancer, spine deterioration, and loss of joint function or mobility can be catastrophic events. These people often need a coach and leader in addition to a physician to manage their condition.

Cultural Conditioning: *A female of Middle-Eastern descent hated the culture from her homeland, but family obligations mandated an arranged marriage. After two children, and physical and emotional abuse caused by her husband, she divorced. Her problems, however, had just begun. Years of abuse had taken their toll on her eyes, and she developed an eye condition. She suffered from Crohn's disease. She was treated for chronic pain of unknown origin for a number of years. Finally, upon arriving at the clinic, she showed symptoms of* *absolute psychological impairment and despair as a result of her day-to-day living with her extended family.*

Her pain exceeded that of most individuals in that the symptoms did not completely correlate with the disease listed in her medical records. She complained of weird bouts of abdominal pain that occasionally, according to the pain, would make her "crazy." My first opinion found the culprit to be severe psychological impairment. During excessively warm periods she would become dehydrated, pass out, and need hospital admission for intravenous hydration and injection of narcotics. This occurred for approximately one and a half years under my care. She had been to ten physicians previously, trying to obtain an overall diagnosis, and had been kicked out of most clinics because of her difficult psychosocial condition and consequent drama. I lent an ear to this individual, suggesting that I understood her plight and her difficulty with convincing the medical establishment that there was something wrong with her.

I listened with cultural diversity in mind, mindful of the typical laws that are expected of a wife in her culture. I was not prejudiced. I shook my head sadly as the facts of her life story unfolded. Different disease states passed through my mind, and at one point I stopped at porphyria.

I remembered from my mentoring physician during my medical school internal medicine rotation that if patients seem absolutely weird, with abdominal pain and neurologic symptoms, to suspect intermittent porphyria.

Of course, who could know that these words, spoken to me twenty-two years ago, would seal a definitive diagnosis of her condition? It became clear that she was not only tortured because of her own culture and its lack of acceptance of her, but also she was tortured because of the medical community's inability to establish a firm diagnosis to characterize her condition.

This often leads to the frustration of patients, namely when a vague diagnosis is offered to them. Before any cure or treatment can begin, a proper diagnosis must be established. This is a fundamental cornerstone of our clinic. Simply put, porphyria is a group of relatively rare disorders that are passed down from families, in which an important part of the hemoglobin, called "hume," is improperly manufactured. It involves three major symptoms: abdominal pain or cramping, light sensitivity causing rashes and scarring of the skin known as photodermatitis, and problems with the nervous system and muscles, including mental disturbances, hysteria, and seizures.

Attacks can occur suddenly, usually with excruciating abdominal pain, followed by vomiting, nausea, and constipation. Occasionally there can be sun sensitivity, with blistering, skin rashes, and swelling. There can be scarring of the skin, with color changes. The urine can be tinged reddish or brown after an acute attack. Other symptoms include personality changes, back pain, pain in the arms and legs, numbness in the extremities, muscle weakness or paralysis, and muscle pain.

Herein lies the difficulty of diagnosis. Most hospital emergency rooms or clinics do not think of porphyria as a condition that will exist, causing these problems. During an acute attack, treatment involves infusion of hemotin given intravenously, and pain medications and sedatives to alleviate the symptoms. Other treatments may include glucose dosages to increase carbohydrate levels, which limit the production of porphyrants in the body. One of the main problems with acute and intermittent porphyria is that in some instances it takes up to seven to nine years to make an accurate diagnosis. Whether this is due to a lack of foundational knowledge in the medical community or to the myriad of symptoms that seem to have no correlation, acute and intermittent porphyria is often underdiagnosed and misdiagnosed.

During the first attack the patient, while under my care, was hospitalized, and urine studies were sent for a suspected porphyria attack. The results were inconclusive initially, and this may have been because of the failure to obtain the urine specimen to assess porphyran levels in a timely fashion.

A second attack, months later, brought another round of confusing data. Some of the urine values in this case indicated high positive porphyrant levels, of which eight or so subtypes were evaluated. The facts that there are various types of porphyrants and that symptoms can be widely varied make the condition hard to diagnose.

Normally, the body makes "hem" part of the hemoglobin molecule in a multistep process. Porphyrants are made during several steps of the process. Patients who have porphyria have a deficiency of an enzyme needed in this process. This causes abnormal amounts of porphyrants to build up in the body. Drugs, infection, dehydration, alcohol, and hormones are known to trigger attacks of certain types of porphyria.

Once diagnosis was made, it was given to the patient and her family. The patient experienced initial relief after learning that an actual disease was causing her pain. Subsequently, this relief changed to disbelief as the family convinced her that the diagnosis was impossible. Again, she wrestled with psychological despair and futility. Since the very nature of the disease can cause permanent scarring and neuropsychiatric symptoms, such patients often feel as though they are losing their minds.

Numerous sessions were set up with our pain psychologist as well as other social workers to convince her that she was not crazy and that indeed she had an identifiable condition. Education and treatment followed. To this day I still treat this individual, but I believe her family still doesn't believe her. Maintaining touch with this patient is important, as often I'll get a call from an emergency room where she has been admitted with an acute attack.

Once I communicate with the admitting doctor, the feelings of helplessness and embarrassment from having to ask for pain medication and intravenous treatment are eliminated. Patients that are this ill do not seek medication unless absolutely necessary to prevent a porphyria attack. They've been instructed to get intravenous fluids and glucose.

Often, they are confused with patients who simply seek "a recreational high." They are labeled as "malingerers," but nothing could be further from the truth. Again, the psychological aspect of a condition treated by a health-care professional who understands the disease leads to greater likelihood of successful treatment and less frequency of attacks.

In addition, the belief system that this patient engendered allowed for the possibility that such a disease could be diagnosed with her. If she was as narrow-minded as her family, a firm diagnosis would have been much more difficult to achieve.

The belief system is a very core principle in establishing a treatment algorithm for chronic pain sufferers. If a person believes that something will not work for them, then it is unlikely that that treatment will be beneficial. If the patient is open-minded, on the other hand, and willing to give the treatment a chance, then it has a chance to help the patient.

Again, I'm going to quote Virgil: "They can if they think they can."

Please refer to the website www.gotpaindocs.com, www.thegreatPainJack.com, or www.thegreatPainJack.org, for further information.

Chapter 16:

New Frontiers of Pain Treatment

P ain management is an evolving science. Chronic pain management deals with the ever-changing trial and error methodology of finding out what works best to treat certain conditions. The information age has truly been a boon for the treatment of pain management patients. Information can be shared rapidly amongst the scientific community and chronic pain sufferers alike.

Through information obtained online, worldwide communication can be promulgated, and free access to treatment programs for rare and difficult to treat conditions can be assumed. For example, certain networks now have the capability of linking the chronic pain sufferer in suburban Nebraska to a qualified pain management practitioner in a nearby city. Likewise, support groups and organizations that specialize in care and treatment recommendations for certain conditions like fibromyalgia and diabetes can provide a valuable resource for patients seeking the right providers.

Recently, I was contacted by an individual who had had three glassopharyngeal nerve microvascular decompression surgeries over the last ten years. She lives in rural Tennessee. These types of theories that may occur through the Internet allow for a rapid transfer of information and referral to the right specialist. The poor woman, who has lost hearing as a result of the surgeries and now has developed a chronic pain syndrome unrelieved by the surgeries, is unable to find a proper treatment for her condition.

Via pain networks we were able to refer her to a proper diagnostic and therapeutic clinic that was close to her home. Scores of queries and searches like this (one hundred thousand to two hundred thousand) are performed each day. It is indeed a boon for chronic pain sufferers to have search mechanisms and reliable social networks available to find care with the proper individual. In the past these individuals would often suffer or be institutionalized without any proper diagnostics or intervention.

Electronic transfer of information, such as texting, may also prove valuable in the future of therapy delivery. For example, a client was referred to me via an attorney six hundred miles away through text messages. The text information was relayed to me as well as images of MRI studies performed on the cervical spine and lumbar spine after a car accident. I was able to access the report and MRI studies and review them thoroughly. The patient was called with regard to her history. After a conversation regarding the care the patient received previously, a full history was then provided.

We had agreed to meet at a surgical center two and a half hours from her home, where we were able to provide the necessary treatment for her. History and physical examination were conducted prior to the procedure, on the day of the service. Prior medical records were phoned in to my office for review. This exemplifies how the electronic transfer of information can assist patients in remote locations, where they may not otherwise find help.

The future of chronic pain management will involve the improvement in imaging studies. Currently, MRI scanners, which operate on a very high Tesla(short for Tera-electronvolt Energy Superconducting Linear Accelerator or the magnetic flux density of a magnet used in a scanner to recreate body images can detect very small abnormalities and defects by having strong magnetic fields, which may provide more reliable data. MRI studies prove to be best for showing spinal cord, nerve, or soft tissue. Ultrasound scanning has improved greatly, and 3D Doppler ultrasound is a noninvasive, cost-effective means for identifying pathology outside the spine. As its improvements continue, it is likely that 3D imaging of the spine will provide superior imaging without the additional cost of MRI studies and the radiation associated with CAT scans.

Diagnostic imaging involving CT scanning will also improve in the future. CAT scans will produce less radiation. For example, at this time if cancer is diagnosed, an oncologist or surgeon may request CAT scans every six months. This is an inordinate amount of REDs and radiation that will perhaps have a toxic effect long-term, especially if the patient is undergoing chemotherapy or immune-suppression therapy. Thin-slice CAT scanning with a pared-down amount of radiation will be indeed important in the future of imaging.

Three-dimensional helical scanners using computerized 3D-reconstruction are also at the forefront of current medical diagnostic testing. This type of scanning is thought to be superior for obtaining imaging of vascular structures that may be difficult to image via traditional studies.

It is likely that a tagging system will be developed for tagging damaged nerve cells. This will be used cooperation with scanning devices that can identify injured tissue and spinal cord damage. If the tagging system can be developed for imaging of spinal motor and sensory tracts that occur like fibers in the spinal cord, this would greatly improve the diagnostic capability of identifying lesions within the spinal cord and peripheral nerves, as well as spinal nerves.

Similarly, CAT scanners or positive emission tomography studies have been used in the brain to identify functional abnormalities. These studies have been used with modest success in identifying disease states that may show functional aberrations in brain mechanisms.

Identifying and tagging damaged nerve cells will then be easier to treat, as these damaged neural tissues will light up on the scanner, and a practitioner will have successfully received the information on specifically where the abnormal nerve cells are.

Drug delivery systems will also be improved in the new horizons of medicine. Specialized products known as liposomes structures are formed by biological cell layers that have a water-attracting molecule on one end and a fat-attracting molecule on the other. When large numbers of these phosphor-lipid molecules are placed in a space, they will raise themselves spontaneously to max their water and fat-loving heads in an organized fashion. These comprise the basis for a cellular membrane.

Medications must be able to permeate the cell membrane and get to its nucleus to have the desired effect. Liposomes, which allow for this type of permeation, are an exciting new advance in drug delivery. Certain medications, including vaccines, antibacterials, and antichemotherapeutic agents can be incorporated into these liposomes to fool the "guards" of the cell membrane and enter the cell.

Likewise, topicals, or medications that are applied to the skin, also can be incorporated into liposome technology. Liposome technology can be dangerous in that during the formation of the active ingredient certain toxins or chemicals can be inadvertently incorporated into the formation of the liposome, making the liposome act like a Trojan horse, sneaking a disease or bacteria into cells.

The danger of the ability of phosphor-lipids to act as the carriers for delivering active ingredients directly into the cell is impressive. Alone, they are nontoxic, but their ability to carry toxic and contaminated substances is where the problem lies. Careful manufacturing of raw materials, the timeliness, and thermal activity during preparation and storage are critically important to their success. The FDA has not decided whether liposome products should be considered a medicine and put under the scrutiny of physicians.

Commonly in practice, for treatment of chronic pain conditions such as fibromyalgia, a liposome mechanism is used in incorporating agents to permeate the skin and the subcutaneous tissues. These delivery vehicles can deliver their payload into far-reaching areas, including inside a damaged osteoarthritic knee.

Research is currently being performed on laser activation of cells treated with prior liposomal activity. The low-intensity laser is a device that activates the midochondrial activity of the cell, thereby increasing its thermal activity. When this happens, enzyme activity increases, which drives cellular processes, causing the cell to heal and reproduce at a faster rate.

Exciting new research using multimodal therapy with liposomal delivery of topical anesthetic and low-intensity laser therapy is being performed. Under way are trials where tissue is activated using the lasers, and liposomal delivery of medication is enhanced after this process. The process of low-intensity laser activating the cells, therefore turning on their thermal activity, and enzyme acceleration can prove to be an exciting new area of improving benefits without surgery or injection therapy.

Commonly, it is accepted in the pain management world that it is difficult to get the drug, whether it be a steroid, anesthetic, or other medicinal, to the area of greatest need. Traditional methods of delivery include injection therapy. If liposomal therapy can successfully be incorporated into topical agents, then needle injections may be a thing of the distant past.

In the future, horizons of treatment of chronic pain patients will involve marking for disease on a preventative basis. An assessment of whether somebody carries a gene for development of diabetes, for example, may change medications prescribed or may include preventative measures to assure prevention of disease.

Likewise, the future may involve a genetic modification or treatment of the genetic code prior to the development of an inherited condition, such as Huntington's chorea. Genetic modification can be used for the treatment of disease or prevention of that disease.

Much research needs to be completed on gene therapy, and a firm understanding of how a genetic code predisposes to the development of disease states such as degenerative disk disease or neurological disorders such as Parkinson's needs to be determined. Perhaps the future will hold a mechanism for disease prevention rather than treatment after the disease has taken hold.

Stem cell research has largely been on hold during the last decade. There are a number of reasons this has occurred. The pluro-potential stem cell, which is the shell that can lead to many different cell lines when placed within an individual, shows exciting promise for treatment of disorders such as disk disease and spinal cord injury.

The placement of an undifferentiated cell (that is to say a cell that has not decided what it wants to be what it grows up) is part impartial to the way stem cells work. An undifferentiated stem cell placed in a tissue that needs regeneration can grow into a new, healthy, viable cell of that particular structure. Research has been thwarted by efforts of some individuals and groups that do not advocate this type of testing for future clinical usage of stem cells derived from embryonic cell lines.

Without espousing any political controversy, it can be expected that stem cells will eventually play an important role in the development and treatment of injured tissue in the chronic pain population. It is up to society to decide when and at what time the clinical research trials using these all-powerful embryonic stem cells occur.

Stem cell research has been ongoing in the field of spinal cord injury. However, mainstream stem cell therapy is another story entirely. In the future, stem cell therapy may indeed be something that will enable our bodies to heal with relative ease. This may occur through blood storage at the time of delivery, whereby the cryogenic freeze of embryonic or fetal cord blood can deliver these stem cell lines.

I am not suggesting that fetal blood be preserved at time of delivery for usage for one's own stem cell development later. I am simply suggesting that options for growing and harvesting living tissue based on stem cell lines is an ideal way to regenerate injured tissue later in an individual's life. Such replications could involve regrowing cartilage in an athlete's degenerated knee, regenerating tendon and cartilage formation in a work-injury shoulder patient, and regenerating cell growth in spinal cord accident quadriplegic patients. The possibilities the future holds are myriad in this type of delivery mechanism in treatment of chronic pain patients.

Wonder Drugs

Because of the relatively easy access to pain medication and higher prescribing rates due to the enhanced recognition rate of chronic pain as a specific medical subspecialty, the problem of dependency and addiction has grown inordinately. This leaves physicians and researchers looking for different types of solutions.

In the last decade there has been recognition of natural compounds occurring in nature and of the enhanced research of the phenomenon of pain on a cellular level in attempts to find new classes of nonaddictive pain medications.

One area of growth of nonaddictive pain medication is the antinerve growth factor antibodies. Antinerve growth factor and the interaction of nerve growth factor on the regeneration of injured tissue have been investigated by a number of researchers. The pharmaceutical company Pfizer developed a new drug that had been shown to be effective in an initial study of patients with osteoarthritis of the knee.

The drug was originally thought to be a nonaddictive biological agent. It specifically is a human monoclonal antibody for nerve growth factor. Nerve growth factor (NGF) plays an essential role in nerve growth and maintenance. When an injury happens, the level of NGF rises in the body and creates generalized pain sensations. The drug was designed to act against NGF to prevent the increase in pain sensations during the injury or in certain diseases.

The drug was unfortunately halted in June 2008 by the FDA; reports surfaced that the drug made the joint condition worse and led to complete joint replacements. This NGF antibody has been tested by Pfizer for diabetic neuropathy and lower back pain. Regeneron Pharmaceuticals and Ortho-McNeill-Janson Pharmaceuticals also have similar products that are in development stages. Both these companies have products in which preliminary testing has indicated that there are significant improvements in patients with osteoarthritis of the knee.

Recent interest has also been surrounding the immobilizing venoms that have been isolated from marine creatures that are scattered along the ocean floor, amongst coral reefs. These creatures for centuries have preyed upon fish, worms, and crustaceans and have used their dangerous venoms to paralyze their prey. The same venom isolated from these marine creatures has been used to help people suffering from chronic pain.

Conotoxins, as they are called, work by isolating certain receptors and sensory nerves and causing a targeting of their activity. Unlike opioids, the conotoxins do not travel through the central nervous system. Conotoxins consist of protein fragments or conopeptides. Prialt (ziconotide) is a synthetic omega conotoxin. This is available and FDA-approved to treat severe to intractable nerve pain.

Ziconotide inhibits presynaptic calcium channels, which means that the toxin affects the calcium release from certain terminals that control nerve function. The drug works by binding to a calcium channel receptor located on pain fibers within the spinal cord. This produces an analgesic effect by inhibiting the firing of sensory fibers entering the part of the spinal cord known as the dorsal laminar of the spinal grey matter.

This ostensibly prevents sensory fibers from sending messages that are pain signals to the brain, preventing the sensation from occurring. Thus, ziconotide seems to be a new class of peptide medications with potent pain-relieving and antiaddictive properties, along with depression of the central nervous system and respiration, making it relatively safe. Unfortunately the drug must be administered intrathecally, into the central spinal system directly.

The study of conotoxins in general has utmost potential to make an impact on the field of pain management. Ziconotide, a derivative conotoxin is one of the few marine-originating medications that targets calcium channels. The challenge will be to find an analog of ziconotide that can be administered through a pill.

Scientists will have to arrange a molecule to pass the brain-blood barrier, since most of the targets of conotoxins are located in the brain. Other research of conopeptides is a molecule that belongs to the chi-conopeptide family and targets the norepinephrine, which is an essential neuron transmitter for neural function. Conotoxins are also being studied for treatment of Alzheimer's disease, addiction medication, Parkinson's disease, multiple sclerosis, and a host of other neurological illnesses.

In addition to conotoxins, the essence of chili peppers and their capsaicins cousins have been studied with great interest in recent years. Researchers at the University of Texas Health Science Center in San Antonio were able to uncover a family of "indigenous capsaicins" that are present in humans and have developed two drugs designed to treat pain.

Capsaicin has been used as an additive in some pain ointments to decrease nerve sensitivity. Chili peppers contain capsaicins that can cause a painful sensation by activating a transient potential banilloid (trpv-1). Thus, natural indigenous capsaicins are formed by pain cells in response to heat or injury.

Doctor Kenneth M. Hargreaves, the lead researcher , has found that these capsaicin molecules effect oxidized linoleic acid metabolites (or OLAMs). By heating the skin or causing tissue injury, the release of OLAMs will activate the trpv-1 receptor.

There are two new classes of drugs then, designed to block the formulation of OLAMs, or to make antibodies that inactivate them. These are considered to be novel and exciting new investigational approaches to treating chronic and acute pain syndromes. There is evidence to suggest that these molecules are involved in many types of pain, including inflammation, cancer pain, burn pain, and other chronic pain conditions.

Drugs that typically block OLAMs may constitute an approach to pain management. Unlike opioids, these drugs do not have a chemical addiction potential. Fortunately, further research is being performed to rapidly push these drugs to market.

It is well known about the addictive properties of opioids. The concept of physiologic dependency is well documented. However, the opioid powerful effect on pain relief cannot be discredited.

Drugs that target glial cells are an attempt to stop tolerance and dependence on medication at the source and keep the *beneficial* effect of opioids intact. Glial cells play an important role in providing support and maintaining healthy function of neurons in the brain. Opioids, including morphine, heroin, and OxyContin, all tend to overactivate glial cells, which then in turn begin to stop the pain suppression properties of the drugs.

Opioids additionally connect with the appropriate receptors but also with the glial cell receptors. This leads to greater tolerance and dependence, affecting the addiction factor. There have been extensive attempts to prevent opioids from stimulating the glial cells in order to deliver the pain relief without the side effects of addiction. Experimental drugs have been created to block morphine's effects on glial cells. Indeed, it may be a glial cell blocker that allows continued usage of opioid medications without the unwanted side effects of addiction.

Glial cells may also have an effect on other aspects of opioid use, such as reward hyperalgesia and tolerance. There may be in fact ways to treat pain with much lower dosage of opioids if glial cells blockers are incorporated into therapy. There also may be the possibility of not having to adjust for tolerance or for serious side effects.

The Centers for Disease Control reported that between 1999 and 2006 the number of poisoning deaths nearly doubled. This is largely because of the deaths following opioid prescription overdose. Yet the usage of these medications remains extremely high because of their absolute effectiveness in pain relief. So the search for nonaddictive drugs for moderate to severe pain is extremely complex.

Postopioid medications target the central nervous system; it is thought by some researchers that the ideal target for a new pain medication or class of pain medications would not use the central nervous system, since that would increase the risk of activating central dopamine systems and produce analgesic tolerance.

Some researchers believe the OLAM system has a key point of interest in this regard. Since opioid receptors are responsible in greatest extent for all of these pain addiction problems, it will be necessary to target a solution to this by looking at the receptors themselves. These are very good painkillers, but tolerance is such a huge problem that people who take medication on a long-term basis may potentially not get any pain relief at all.

Ziconotide is the first major painkiller approved by the FDA in the past twenty-five years that is a nonnarcotic. It would be thus impossible to develop an addiction to ziconotide, because it works by a different mechanism. Ziconotide blocks neural transmission instead of blocking the receptors that are the target in addiction syndrome.

In the central nervous system, opioids and other medications can unintentionally produce side effects including dry mouth, constipation, and sensory effects that can alter the perception of pain. It is likely possible to counteract these unwanted side effects using some kind of dual therapy that will limit the possibility of developing tolerance and the potential for addiction. This concept of dual therapy will maximize safety and efficacy of the medication.

Summing up, whether the concept of blocking the transmission of pain signals (by targeting certain substances), blocking the glial cells in order to maximize the pain relieving effect of opioids, or using genetic or genomic sequencing to knock out certain chemicals in the manifestation of pain, the goals are the same: to offer effective pain relief without the possibility for addiction and dependency. Coupled with the ability to provide diagnostic and often therapeutic injection therapy, this dynamic combination of injectable medication options as well as perhaps ingested medication options will serve to fundamentally alter the way that pain management is practiced into the future. It is clear that the chronic pain condition will not likely go away at any point in the near future for afflicted individuals. It is the art and science of blending these exciting new methods of delivery options in treating chronic pain that will diminish the human suffering component and also allow for the decreased potential for harmful and addictive medications to control the will of the afflicted individual.

About the Author

Dr John F. Petraglia is a board-certified anesthesiologist and pain management specialist practicing in Southern California and the Central Valley of California. He shares his greater than twenty-five-year experience of treating chronic and acute pain conditions through the eyes of a busy pain management provider. He provides information relating to proper diagnosis and includes sketches and workbook type questionnaires in an effort to help the reader better understand and work with his or her physician to diagnose their condition. Dr. Petraglia shares these stories of chronic pain affliction through the vignettes of characters that may suffer similar conditions in order to provide learning and direction to the reader. Dr. Petraglia attended medical school at the State University of New York at Downstate Medical Center and performed his residency at the New York Hospital Cornell-Columbia Medical Center. He currently has an active practice in all aspects of pain management, is published in medical journals, and is involved in weekly support group education to help those who suffer with chronic pain better understand the proper usage of medications.

List Of Research Material

http://www.gotpaindocs.com interventional pain medical group website

http://www.greatpainjack.com about the great pain jack

http://www.asipp.org/about_us.html American society of interventional pain physicians

www.getnulooks.com cosmetic treatment can help chronic pain

www.wantnulooks.com healing the body and the mind through the outside and inside

http://www.asahq.org
American society of Anesthesiologists

http://www.doctorsforpain.com/ finding a pain clinic

http://www.painmed.org
American Academy of Pain Medicine

http://www.fibromyalgia.com Fibromyalgia

http://www.fibromyalgia-support.org/ fibromyalgia treatment

http://www.spinaldiagnostics.com/sdx/_SDPhysicians/SDPhysicians.asp?id=Dr_Derby
pain practice doctor website

http:/ /nccam.nih.gov /health/meditation/ overview.htm
national center for complementary and alternative medicine

http://www.bcia.org/ biofeedback certification institute of America

http://aath.org/ - association for applied and therapeutic humor

http://www.aapb.org/ -association for applied psychophysiology and biofeedback

http:/ /www.natboard.com/ national board for certified clinical hypnotherapists

http://www.cure-back-pain.org/psychologically-induced-pain-syndromes.html
-list of psychologically induced pain syndromes

http://www.healingchronicpain.org/content/introduction/conv_ mndbdy.asp

types of psychological/ mind-body therapies, including hypnosis, prayer, etc

http://psychologyofpain. blogspot.com/ -psychology of pain blog

http://www.nationalpainfoundation.org/articles/703/psychological-factors-and-pain
National Pain Foundation's site on psychological factors and pain

http://my.clevelandclinic.org/disorders/back_ pain/hic_psychological_ factors _of_ chronic_ back_ pain.aspx
psychological factors of chronic back pain

http://www.healthpsych.com/bhi/glossary.pdf
-glossary of terms relating to psychological factors in pain

http://paincenter.stanford.edu/patient _care/therapy.html
Stanford pain center site on psychological treatment for pain
cultural responses to pain management

http:/ /pediatric-pain.ca/professional/internationalForum/Finley. pdf
powerpoint presentation on cultural perceptions of pain management

http://www.thenewageblog.com/hypnotherapy-in-the-treatment-of-phantom-pain/
article on the use of hypnotherapy in treating phantom pain

http:/ /www.ncbi.nlm.nih.gov/pmc/articles/PMC 1276504/
essay on cross-cultural perspectives on pain

http:/ /www.health.com/health/condition-article/0,,20222981,00.html
index of websites dealing with particular aspects of alternative approaches to pain management

http://www. webmd.com/pain-management/ guide/pain-management -alternative-therapy article on alternative pain therapies

http://www.biofeedbacktherapy.net/
page dedicated to biofeedback therapy/

http://www. umm.edu/news/releases/ alternative   therapies.htm
alternative methods of managing shock trauma

http://www.pamelaegan.com/articles/pain-management-chart.htm
alternative pain management therapy chart

http://healing.about.com/od/energyhealing/a/energy spsmith.htm
article on energy healing

http://www.skepdic.com/essays/energyhealing.htm
article on energy healing

http://www.umassmed.edu/content.aspx?id=41252

"The **Center for Mindfulness in Medicine, Health Care, and Society** is a visionary force and global leader in mind-body medicine. For thirty years, we have pioneered the integration of mindfulness meditation and other mindfulness-based approaches in mainstream medicine and healthcare through patient care, research, academic medical and professional education, and into the broader society through diverse outreach and public service initiatives."

http://illinoispain.com/news/cbpainmedicine.pdf
New Frontiers in Community Pain Medicine

http://www. webmd.com/pain-management/ guide/pain-relief-without–pills
-article on pain relief without use of pills (acupuncture, etc)

http://www. webmd.com/pain-management/tc/chronic-pain-other-treatment
alternative treatments for chronic pain (acupuncture, biofeedback, hypnosis, etc)

http://www.mentalhealthmatters.com/index.php?option=com_content&view=article&id=425 -10 tips for mental pain relief

http:/ /www.ehow.com/about_5563224_cultural-responses-pain-management.html
–cultural responses to pain management

http://www.healthpsych.com/bhi/glossary.pdf
good glossary of terms relating to psychological factors in pain

http://pediatric-pain.ca/professional/internationalForum/Finley.pdf
-presentation on cultural perceptions of pain management

http://www.ncbi.nlm.nih.gov/pmc/articles/PMC1276504/
essay on cross- cultural perspectives on pain

Pain-Wise -A Patient's guide to Pain Management –David Kloth, MD_hatherleigh Press N. Y. 2011

The Use of Botulinum Toxin Type A in Pain Management second edition Martin K. Childers D.O. mic Information Systems 2002

A guide to physical examination third edition Barbara Bates, M.D. JB Lippincott company, Philadelphia 1983

Interventional pain management second edition Stephen D. Waldman, M.D., JD WB Saunders Company , New York 2001

Neurological differential diagnosis John Patton 1983 Harold Starke Ltd. London

The pain practitioner volume 20 number four Winter 2010

Pain physician volume 13 number 6 December 2010

Occupational medicine practice guidelines second edition evaluation and management of common health problems and functional recovery and workers leg as glass, M.D. OEM press Beverly Farms, Massachusetts 2004

Management of acute and chronic neck pain and evidence-based approach Nicolai Bogduk, Brian McGuirk Elsevier , 2006

Ageless body, timeless mind -a quantum alternative to growing old Deepak Chopra, M.D. Harmony books, New York 1993

The truth about chronic pain patients and professionals on how to face it, understand it, overcome it Arthur Rosenfeld M.D. basic books, 2003

Injection techniques in orthopedic and sports medicine Stephanie Saunders second edition WB Saunders Edinburg 2002

Orthopedic examination, evaluation, and intervention second edition Mark Dutton, PT McGraw-Hill medical New York 2008

Neurological differential diagnosis Mark Mumenthaler, M.D. Thieme-Stratton Inc. New York 1985

Regional block - a handbook for use in clinical practice of medicine and surgery Daniel C. Moore, M.D. Josie Thomas publisher Springfield Illinois 1953

Healthy Healing-an alternative Healing reference Linda C. Rector-P age, M.D., PhD ninth edition June 1992

The Healing Herbs the ultimate guide to the curative power of natures medicines Michael Castleman Rodale press, Pennsylvania 1991

Adrenal fatigue the 21st-century stress syndrome James L. Wilson, M.D., DC, PhD Smart publications , Petaluma California 2007

Just fine - unmasking concealed chronic illness and pain Carol Sveilich, MA Avid Reader press, Austin Texas 2005

Informational You tube video channels :
"the pain doctors"

"Beyond pain management"
"Dr. John Petraglia"

http://www.youtube.com/user/drjohnpetraglia?feature=mhum#p/a/u/1/
> xFts0CabJqg

> http://www.youtube.com/user/drjohnpetraglia?feature=mhum#p/a/u/1/
> xFts0CabJqg

http://abclocal.go.com/kfsn/story?section=news/health/health_watch&id=6142110
treating painful cellulite him and

http://www.youtube.com/user/gotpaindocs

http://www.youtube.com/user/johnpetraglia

http://www.youtube.com/user/painmanagementbeyond

http://www.youtube.com/user/thepaindoctors

http://www.youtube.com/user/drjohnpetraglia

http://www.youtube.com/user/greatpainjack

http://www.getnulooks.com/

http://www.gotpaindocs.com/